natural remedies
for morning sickness and other
pregnancy
problems

natural remedies
for morning sickness and other
pregnancy
problems

Denise Tiran

Quadrille

First published in 2001 by
Quadrille Publishing Limited
Alhambra House
27-31 Charing Cross Road
London WC2H 0LS

Editorial Director Jane O'Shea
Art Director Mary Evans
Designer Jim Smith
Editor Sarah Widdicombe
Production Julie Hadingham

Illustrations Bridget Bodoano

Cataloguing in Publication Data: a catalogue record for this book
is available from the British Library.

ISBN 1 902757 88 2
Printed and bound by Mackays of Chatham, England.

contents

 self help and complementary care 8

 therapies and remedies 18

 symptoms and discomforts of pregnancy 68

 illness in pregnancy 112

 the birth 144

 mother and baby 176

self-help and complementary care

Congratulations – you're pregnant! Now that you have overcome some of the surprise, or even shock, that you are soon to be a mother, you will be wondering how you can do the best for your baby and how to prepare yourself for the birth and parenthood. I hope that you will be enjoying your pregnancy, but you may be unfortunate enough to be suffering some of the many aches, pains and other discomforts that can occur during this time. You may be worrying about the birth itself and wondering how you will cope with your contractions. The thought of parental responsibility may also be overwhelming.

You will no doubt have been told that, where possible, you should avoid taking any medications during pregnancy, especially in the first three months when all of your baby's major organs are developing, in order to reduce the risk of abnormalities. In any case, I am sure that you would like to keep your pregnancy as normal as possible, with only as much medical intervention as is essential. You may already have considered the use of natural remedies to resolve some of your discomforts but may be unsure about their safety during pregnancy. The very fact that you have picked up this book hopefully indicates that you have an interest in complementary therapies and wish to find out more about how they work, whether or not they are safe and where to find them.

This book is intended to provide you with sufficient information to make informed choices about whether or not you would like to use aspects of complementary therapies during your pregnancy, the birth of your baby and in the weeks that follow. The emphasis is on the safe and appropriate incorporation of the therapies into the care which you will also be receiving from the conventional maternity services in your area. Some of the suggestions you can administer yourself, for others you will need to seek expert help from a practitioner. Throughout, I have used practical examples from my own complementary therapy midwifery clinic (although minor details and names have been changed) to illustrate what can be done.

I hope you will enjoy reading the book and will find the ideas and suggestions for using complementary therapies both informative and helpful. Whatever you decide to do, I hope you experience a happy and enjoyable pregnancy, and I wish you well for the birth of your new baby.

what is complementary and alternative medicine?

Complementary and alternative medicine is any form of healthcare that falls outside the mainstream provision of conventional medicine. Orthodox healthcare in the western world involves the use of drugs, surgery and occasionally specialist techniques such as radiotherapy, but very rarely incorporates acupuncture, reflexology or other complementary therapies. However, in other areas of the world such as Asia these techniques are used alongside so-called conventional medicine and they are certainly not regarded as alternative.

The term 'alternative' implies that these techniques are selected *instead* of the more normally prescribed medicines or operative procedures, and indeed there may be situations where it is appropriate to consult a practitioner of one of these therapies rather than a doctor – for example, osteopathy or chiropractic may be a more effective treatment for a bad back than physiotherapy or surgery. Many people refer to 'natural' medicine, specifically in relation to therapies such as herbal medicine, aromatherapy and homeopathy, but it is important, particularly in maternity care when both you and your baby are receiving the treatment, to remember that 'natural' does not necessarily mean 'safe'. All complementary therapies must be used appropriately – if they are powerful enough to treat various ailments positively, then they can also be potent enough, if used incorrectly, potentially to do harm. On the other hand, 'complementary' suggests that whatever therapy is chosen it is used in conjunction with conventional care, to enhance and support the treatment already provided, such as using acupuncture for pain relief after an operation.

There is a great deal of interest among the public in the use of complementary and alternative medicine, with about one in three people in the UK and up to 50 per cent in the USA having used one or more therapies. Consequently, there is an increasing demand for them to be made more readily available. Health professionals are also becoming much more interested and involved in using the therapies in conjunction with their normal practice, and there is a move towards greater integration of complementary with conventional medicine. What originally began as 'fringe medicine' – or even 'witchcraft' – has become increasingly accepted and steadily incorporated into healthcare facilities in the western world.

All complementary and alternative therapies have an underlying philosophy of 'holism' – in other words, they view the whole person as a distinct individual, and focus on the way in which the body, mind and spirit all interact with one another. It has only been in recent years that doctors have, for example, recognized the physical effects which severe emotional stress can have, such as raising blood pressure or leading to heart attacks. Similarly, serious physical ill health can have a detrimental effect on the emotional and spiritual sides of an individual's life.

Another aspect of complementary medicine is the partnership between the practitioner and the client. If you visit a complementary therapist you may be given advice to help you adjust your diet or lifestyle, such as taking more exercise, and will be seen as a partner in achieving better health, with the professional being a facilitator. Frequently you will experience a 'healing crisis' when you first start the treatment as your body 'kick starts' itself into getting better. This means that you may initially feel worse before you begin to improve, but this is normal. It is a measure of the power of the different therapies that you may experience this apparently negative effect, but very soon you should start to see a change for the better.

safety and efficacy

There are over 200 therapies which may be considered to be complementary or alternative, but only about 15–20 have credibility at present. That is not to say that the remainder are ineffective, but currently there is insufficient evidence to demonstrate their safety. Throughout the medical professions there is a great clamour for care to be based on the evidence of research, and this applies as much to complementary as to orthodox medicine. For years there has been plenty of anecdotal evidence that various therapies are effective, but in order for them to be accepted by doctors large-scale trials need to be undertaken. Some therapies are better researched than others: for example, acupuncture for sickness has been studied in many centres, and aromatherapy trials have proved that essential oils are effective at combating infections.

This need for evidence extends to demonstrating not only the effectiveness of a therapy but also its safety. Obviously patients and clients want to know that whatever care they are given is safe, and with so many legal cases involving healthcare, doctors also want to be sure, almost beyond doubt, that providing complementary therapies will not knowingly cause harm. This means that complementary and alternative medicine has to prove itself virtually twice over in order for the medical profession to accept it, which is laudable but unrealistic – and somewhat unfair when you consider that much of conventional medicine was introduced without trials to prove its safety. It is, however, this perceived lack of evidence which causes many doctors to adopt a sceptical and sometimes antagonistic attitude towards complementary therapies.

Denigration of complementary therapies is, thankfully, diminishing, and this is largely due to the fact that the complementary medical professions are themselves acknowledging the need for research. In addition, the recognition that many therapies produce results and improve the general well-being of clients is very much in their favour at a time when healthcare consumers feel dissatisfied with much of the conventional health services. Also, the education and training of complementary practitioners is delivered to a much higher academic level than was previously the case, with many therapies requiring students to achieve degrees in the relevant subject.

The therapies which are most widely accepted are also the most sophisticated and well developed in terms of training and regulation of practitioners and research. There are five therapies that are complete systems of medicine in their own right: osteopathy, chiropractic, homeopathy, acupuncture and herbal medicine. Other therapies such as aromatherapy, reflexology, massage, shiatsu and hypnotherapy are more supportive therapies, usually used alongside one of the main five or in conjunction with conventional healthcare; they are also those therapies which are commonly considered to be primarily of benefit for relaxation, although this is by no means their only value.

complementary therapies in maternity care

Complementary therapies can be of enormous help during pregnancy, childbirth and early parenthood. Often the therapies are viewed simply as a means of aiding relaxation and it can be very beneficial to receive regular therapy such as aromatherapy, massage or reflexology throughout pregnancy. However, complementary therapies can also be used to ease specific discomforts of pregnancy, reduce pain in labour and assist with some of the minor complications which may occur as your body returns to the non-pregnant state after the birth. This is really where natural therapies come into their own, as they are an invaluable means of enhancing and complementing the standard maternity care that you receive. Indeed, in many countries any care that is provided for pregnant and childbearing women must, by law, be complementary to conventional care, as it is illegal for anyone other than a midwife or doctor, or one in training, to take sole responsibility for maternity care, except in an emergency.

One report in the UK in 1997 suggested that about 34 per cent of midwives have used some form of complementary therapy in their practice. This is primarily in response to demands from pregnant women and their families, who wish to regain control of the child-bearing process, which over the second half of the twentieth century became extremely medicalized. Many women have, in any case, already used complementary medicine, either for themselves or for their families; once they are pregnant, it is a natural progression to use the therapies to deal with problems for which conventional drugs may not be suitable, due to the risk to the unborn baby.

You may come into contact with complementary therapies in a variety of ways:

- You may already have been consulting a therapist, for example a homeopath, prior to becoming pregnant and wish to continue to visit them during your pregnancy.

- You may wish to attend for regular relaxing treatment to help you cope with the stresses and strains of pregnancy.
- You may choose to use some of the natural remedies to ease the discomforts of early pregnancy, especially when you are unable to take conventional medicines.
- You may wish to attend specific antenatal classes to learn how to use one complementary therapy to help you during labour.
- You may choose to have a complementary practitioner with you during labour to act as a birth companion and provide natural methods of pain relief.
- You may – if you are lucky – be offered referral to a complementary therapist within the conventional maternity services.
- Your doctor, midwife or maternity nurse may use one or more therapies as part of the normal care they provide.

If you choose to seek help from a complementary practitioner you should ensure that they are aware that you are pregnant, although most will take a detailed history from you in any case. It should also be stressed that when major complications of pregnancy or labour arise you should be guided by your obstetrician, midwife or maternity nurse as to the most appropriate treatment necessary.

finding a complementary practitioner

If you decide to consult a practitioner of one or more complementary therapies while you are pregnant, you need to be sure that they are well trained and appropriately experienced. It is often difficult to know whether or not this is the case, particularly in countries where regulation of practitioners is not mandatory except for osteopathy and chiropractic, although this situation is gradually changing.

Practitioners of the 'top five' complementary therapies – osteopathy, chiropractic, acupuncture, homeopathy and herbal medicine – will have undergone lengthy programmes of training at a high academic and professional level, and you can be reasonably well assured that they will be able to provide appropriate care, although you should ask what experience they have gained since qualifying in treating pregnant and childbearing women. Many of these practitioners will also be doctors, nurses, midwives or physiotherapists, and although this does not necessarily make them any more competent as complementary therapists, they will already be bound by the professional and disciplinary codes of their original healthcare training.

Similarly, practitioners of some of the supporting therapies outside the 'top five' may also be qualified in another health profession and you may prefer to consult someone who is also a midwife, or you may be fortunate enough to have a midwife in your area who practises a specific therapy. Word of mouth is always a good means of finding a practitioner who is sympathetic, professional, competent, effective and safe. Simply looking up someone in the local telephone directories is not a wise idea – often those therapists with the largest or most eye-catching advertisements are those most desperate for business! Your midwife or family doctor may be able to recommend a suitable practitioner to you.

It may be helpful to ask some of the following questions when you initially consult a practitioner for complementary therapy during pregnancy. If the therapist is unable or unwilling to divulge this information, you should consider whether or not you wish to continue to visit him/her.

- Where and when did you train?
- To which professional register do you belong?
- What professional indemnity insurance cover do you have?
- What courses and further training have you undergone since qualifying?
- What experience do you have of caring for pregnant and childbearing women?
- How much do consultations cost, and how does this compare with other therapists?
- How many visits am I likely to require? (If receiving treatment for a specific problem rather than just relaxation.)
- Will you be liaising with my family doctor and/or midwife?

Tips for a safe and satisfying pregnancy

It is sometimes difficult to take on board all the advice and information you are given about your pregnancy, both from professionals and from friends and family. Health professionals often provide almost *too much* information, sometimes in language that is hard to understand. Alternatively, if they are extremely busy they may not provide adequate explanations regarding matters which you consider important. Occasionally, your midwife, family doctor or obstetrician may give advice or make suggestions for treatment based on their expert judgement, which you do not fully understand or with which you disagree. On the other hand, family members and friends are always keen to tell you about their own childbirth experiences, and often focus on the 'horror stories' they have heard.

Do remember that this is *your* pregnancy: for some women, it is the only one. Pregnancy is a time of great physical and emotional upheaval and you may not always be able to think objectively about what is happening to you. There are, however, many ways in which you can help yourself to achieve the best possible pregnancy and most satisfying labour, and to look forward to the first days with your newborn baby.

- Always ask questions and seek clarification about things that you do not fully understand.
- Write down any questions you may wish to ask your midwife or obstetrician before you see them so that you do not forget.
- Ask your partner or a friend to accompany you to antenatal appointments, so that they can listen to any explanations given and act as your advocate if necessary.
- Be assertive without becoming confrontational, but at the same time listen to the advice given by your doctor and midwife. They aim to act only in your best interests – and remember, they are human too!
- Avoid listening to 'old wives' tales', which can cause anxiety and unnecessary alarm – and are usually embellished for effect!
- Think about when you intend to stop working – if this is your first baby, avoid the temptation to work right up to the due date. Enjoy a few weeks for yourself, because you will *never* have this freedom to do things spontaneously again!
- Try to find 10–15 minutes every day to spend doing something you *want* to do, not something you *have* to do.

- When your baby has arrived, you will be confronted by lots of opinionated 'experts'. Identify *one* person – a friend or a health professional – whose opinions and commonsense you value, and turn to them when you want advice or simply a 'sounding board' for your concerns.
- Prioritize the various things you need to do each day – caring for your baby, yourself, your partner and other family members, your pets, and last of all, tackling the housework!
- Cooking meals, keeping clean and having enough clothes for everyone are priorities – but do you really have to iron the bed sheets or vacuum the floor every day? If necessary, *ask for help*.
- Remember: above all, you do not have to be a *perfect* parent – you only have to be a *good enough* parent.

2

therapies
and remedies

This chapter introduces the main complementary therapies which are currently available and explains how they can be of use during pregnancy and childbirth. General information is given about each therapy, together with a description of what to expect when you visit a practitioner. The ways in which each therapy may be used to help make you more comfortable during pregnancy, labour and early parenthood are discussed and, where possible, there is reference to research into that particular therapy to provide you with information to support its use. Safety considerations are also covered, to help you when visiting a practitioner, or when you wish to administer some of the natural remedies to yourself or to explain to your midwife or doctor what you are doing.

Osteopathy

Osteopathy is a system of complementary medicine based on the principle that the whole body is directly or indirectly linked to the musculoskeletal system. The therapy is concerned with maintaining or restoring the correct interrelationship and balance of the nerves, muscles and skeleton in order to achieve optimum health and well-being. This is done by manual manipulation of the body, focusing specifically on bones, ligaments and joints. Cranial osteopathy, sometimes called craniosacral therapy, involves the very gentle manipulation of the head and sacrum.

There is a very fine balance between all the systems of the body, but this can be disturbed by alterations caused by poor posture, accidents, trauma or previous operations. Misalignment of one area of the body can lead to problems elsewhere; for example, stress and tension in the neck could trigger tensions in the brain and upset the fine balance of hormones released from there and from the ovaries which regulate the female menstrual cycle.

Osteopaths will always consider the person as a whole, not just the symptoms which are causing problems. The osteopath aims to preserve the balance between all areas of the body in order to allow it to function effectively. Most people seem to think that osteopaths deal only with problems such as backache, neck pain or joint problems, but this is not so. Many other conditions respond well to osteopathic treatment, and some research has already been conducted on using osteopathy for women with menopausal symptoms or premenstrual syndrome; stomach ulcers have also been treated successfully.

Osteopathy in pregnancy and childbirth

Pregnancy puts additional strain on the physical body because of the increased weight, changes in posture and effects of the hormones which relax joints, muscles and ligaments. It is feasible to receive regular osteopathy during pregnancy as a means of relieving or even preventing some of the physical symptoms which can occur, although most women would visit a therapist only when problems arise.

Obviously conditions such as backache, headaches and neck pain will respond well to treatment, sciatica particularly so. Other problems such as pregnancy sickness, heartburn, carpal tunnel syndrome (wrist tingling), constipation and swollen ankles can also be relieved. Breathlessness in later pregnancy may be alleviated by the correction of posture through osteopathic treatment, as may those problems which arise from the increasing weight – for example, knee, hip or pelvic pain, including the quite severe pain that some women experience in the pubic bone. Occasionally, discomfort occurs in the coccyx (tailbone), especially when there has been a fracture in earlier years, and osteopathy may help with this problem both prior to labour and afterwards. Osteopathic treatment is also helpful for women who are planning to conceive, in that it assists in realigning the spine and skeleton prior to conception.

Having an osteopath present during labour can be helpful in easing some of the pain of contractions, which may be made worse by severe backache if the baby's head is facing backwards in the mother's pelvis. Following the birth, many osteopaths advocate a visit to ensure that your skeleton is not out of alignment as a result of the position assumed during labour and delivery. Back and neck problems can persist in the early days following the birth if your position for feeding the baby, especially if you are breastfeeding, is not well supported. The baby can also be examined by the osteopath to ensure that s/he has a well developed skeleton and full range of movements.

What to expect from a visit to an osteopath

Most osteopaths do not treat pregnant women exclusively, but will almost always agree to treat you during your pregnancy even if this is not their speciality; a few practitioners specialize in treating expectant and newly delivered women and their babies. However, no osteopath will agree to see you unless you are also receiving regular conventional maternity care.

At your first visit you will be asked to provide a comprehensive medical history, including details about your occupation and lifestyle which may have a bearing on your physical condition. Information about past pregnancies and the current one to date will also be required. You will then be asked to undress to your underwear and the osteopath will carry out a visual examination of your spine and skeleton. This includes looking at the way you stand, your weight distribution between your two legs, and whether any adaptation in posture is causing extra strain on muscles or ligaments. The osteopath will then feel your spinal column and assess any areas which may indicate possible problems, and will ask you to perform a range of movements of your arms, legs and back. You will be assessed in a sitting position and then lying on the couch, both on your back and, if possible, on your front. Other tests of your reflexes may also be carried out.

Once the osteopath has finished the initial examination and a diagnosis has been made, your treatment will be planned and may include special massage techniques to soften up the muscles before more specific osteopathic movements are made. Osteopathy is not painful, although it can be uncomfortable at times – and occasionally you may be surprised by cracking sounds as your joints are manipulated! Treatment may be weekly or every other week at first, but may then be offered at regular monthly intervals up to and following delivery. Most treatment will be given while you lie on your side with your abdomen supported on a pillow, or you may be asked to sit up for some parts of the process. Your partner may be invited to accompany you in later pregnancy in order to be shown some simple techniques to help you during labour.

Precautions

It is important to choose an osteopath who is well qualified and preferably experienced in treating women during pregnancy. In most countries, the law requires osteopaths to be registered with a regulatory organization, which will automatically mean that they have undergone an approved training programme.

Osteopathy is safe throughout almost the full duration of pregnancy, although some practitioners will decline to treat you at about 16 weeks, when some major hormonal upheavals are occurring in your body. You should always inform your midwife and doctor that you are receiving osteopathic treatment.

Chiropractic

Chiropractic is a science that is concerned with the relationship of the nervous system to the mechanical system – skeleton, joints, ligaments and muscles – of the body. Although chiropractic principles appear to have been in use for many centuries, modern chiropractic originated in the USA in 1895 and has become the third most commonly used system of medicine in the world today, after conventional medicine and dentistry.

Chiropractic is similar to osteopathy, and indeed developed as an 'offshoot' of this therapy. However, it is more concerned with the relative positions of joints, especially those in the spine, than with their relative mobility. Often, X-rays are used before and after treatment to illustrate the changes that have taken place as a result of the manipulations, although X-rays will not be used during pregnancy. Chiropractors focus more on spinal joints than others, and less massage is used than in osteopathy; different techniques are employed and the practitioner works more directly on the joint to be treated than perhaps on a different part of the body.

Chiropractic in pregnancy and childbirth

The aims of chiropractic treatment during pregnancy are to improve the position and mobility of the spine and pelvis, prevent or treat any muscle, joint or spinal problems which occur, encourage a sense of well-being in the mother and promote a healthy environment in which the baby can grow. The treatment will also prepare the mother for labour and delivery, and enable the body to work at its best at this time; care after the birth helps the mother's body to recover and return to its non-pregnant state.

Back problems such as low back pain, sciatica, chest and rib pain, and neck discomfort can all be helped by chiropractic treatment. Headaches and migraines which are a result of tension on neck muscles and vertebrae may be alleviated; carpal tunnel syndrome (wrist tingling) responds well. Research in the early 1990s found that 84 per cent of women who received chiropractic treatment during pregnancy experienced relief of back pain in labour; interestingly, two research trials found that chiropractic treatment during labour actually reduced the length of the labour.

One of the main problems in pregnancy which responds extremely well to chiropractic is pain in the pubic bone area (symphysis pubis diastasis), and ongoing research seems to support the anecdotal evidence. Another condition involves the tension that pregnancy puts on the sacroiliac joint at the back of the pelvis and there is research which shows chiropractic to be effective in relieving this. In the UK and the USA, some work is being done on the position adopted by the baby, its effects on the mother's spine and pelvis, and how chiropractic treatment and postural changes in the mother can be of use in facilitating the best position for the baby.

What to expect from a visit to a chiropractor

A visit to a chiropractor is similar to one to an osteopath in that a full history is taken, followed by a visual and manual examination and assessment before physical treatment is commenced. Manipulations should be gentle but specific and joints are encouraged to move by special low-amplitude movements made by the practitioner. This helps to reduce any misalignment of your bones, muscles and joints and to restore proper functioning to the affected area. The treatment is usually painless, although the area being worked may feel sensitive. Treatment is performed with you sitting up, lying on your front in early pregnancy and, later, on your side.

Precautions

As with osteopathy, practitioners of chiropractic should be registered with the national regulatory body of the country in which they work. X-rays should not normally be used during pregnancy, so it is wise to check with your chiropractor that they do not intend to use them. Some of the treatment may be performed with you lying on your back, but in late pregnancy this can cause dizziness and a temporarily reduced oxygen supply to the baby, so if you are concerned you should ask to sit up again as soon as possible or to be treated in a sitting position.

Homeopathy

Homeopathy is a system of complementary medicine which treats the whole person and is based on the principle that a minute amount of a substance which, in large doses, might actually *cause* a problem, can in fact be used to *treat* that same problem. The founder of homeopathy was Samuel Hahnemann (1755–1845), a doctor who investigated the fact that Peruvian bark (from which quinine, a drug used to treat malaria, is derived) seemed to bring on the symptoms of malaria in someone who did not have the disease, yet these symptoms disappeared when the Peruvian bark was no longer taken. This led to his theory that 'like cures like' and he found many other substances which worked in a similar way.

This approach contrasts directly with orthodox medicine, which works on the principle of treating with 'opposites' to suppress symptoms. For example, constipation will be treated by a doctor with a medicine which may produce diarrhoea, whereas a homeopath would prescribe a substance which would cause constipation if given in its original form but treats it when given in minute doses. Consider the effects of drinking a lot of strong coffee late at night, which often causes headaches, irritability and an inability to get to sleep: a homeopath would treat someone who presented with insomnia accompanied by headaches and irritability with a homeopathic (ie minute) dose of coffea, made from coffee. Ipecacuanha is known to make people vomit, but in pregnancy it may be used in a minute dose to treat certain types of sickness.

Although many of the homeopathic remedies are given in tablet form, they do not work in the same way as conventional drugs or medicines. It is believed that the remedies contain an energy force which is released from the original substance during the production of the homeopathic tablet by a vigorous shaking called 'succussing'. When a remedy is formulated, the original substance is tested on healthy volunteers to obtain a picture of what symptoms an overdose will cause: this is called 'proving' and is a means of identifying exactly which set of symptoms can be treated with the homeopathic version of the substance. The original substance is then diluted and succussed, and the process is repeated many times: the more dilute the eventual remedy, the more potent it is.

All this means that doctors of conventional medicine can be very sceptical about homeopathy unless they are also trained in this system, because they find it difficult to understand. Homeopathy is, however, a very powerful system of healthcare in its own right and people do not have to believe in it for it to be effective. Indeed, veterinary homeopathy is very popular and effective, and it is not possible to ask an animal if it believes in the treatment given!

It is, however, inappropriate to think that the remedies will do no harm simply because they are diluted doses of the original substance. If someone takes the wrong remedy for too long, it is likely to work in reverse and actually begin to cause the symptom it is intended to treat: this is called 'reverse proving'. This is particularly relevant in pregnancy, and it is therefore important to ensure that the correct remedy is used at all times.

Homeopathic remedies are derived from plants (eg chamomilla, arnica montana, belladonna), animals (eg apis from the bee, sepia from the cuttle fish), minerals (eg silica, phosphorus) and some from disease products (eg tuberculum, diphtherium) and healthy tissues and secretions (eg thyroid). Recent research has investigated the use of a homeopathic remedy made from chocolate to treat obesity, and other remedies are in the process of being devised from granite, hydrogen and scorpion.

Homeopathy in pregnancy and childbirth

In homeopathic terms, pregnancy, labour and birth are considered to be a relatively short-term or 'acute' condition and a period which lends itself admirably to treatment with a small range of homeopathic remedies. Homeopathy seems to work by triggering the body's own natural self-healing capacity and therefore, if used appropriately, should be extremely safe at this time. The remedies will not interact with drugs, although some prescribed medications may antidote the remedies (ie prevent them from working effectively). They will not cause complications of pregnancy such as miscarriage, haemorrhage or problems in labour, and can be self-administered by the mother (probably with some direction from a qualified homeopath).

When considering using homeopathic remedies during pregnancy, it is necessary to be as exact as possible about the nature of the symptoms in order that the correct remedy can be selected. Two women suffering from pregnancy sickness may be given two different remedies because the nature of their nausea and vomiting is different. However, there are a few remedies which are commonly used for many women with the same problems: arnica, for example, is well known as a universal aid to ease bruising, especially after the birth or following Caesarean section. Many women respond to pulsatilla for haemorrhoids; this remedy has also been used to turn breech babies to head-first. Some mothers find that caulophyllum will start labour contractions (but this remedy must be administered carefully and only to appropriately selected mothers). During labour, chamomilla may be used to help a woman who is irritable and cannot cope with the pain or with being touched, and chamomilla granules can ease the discomfort of teething in babies.

A range of conditions which arise in pregnancy and labour can be treated with homeopathy including heartburn, backache, insomnia, carpal tunnel syndrome (wrist tingling) and others. In labour, pain, emotional and physical discomfort, and slow progress can all be treated. Breastfeeding difficulties may be eased, and the baby may respond to homeopathy for colic or constipation. Emergency situations which may arise in labour, such as haemorrhage or the baby failing to breath adequately at birth, can be treated with homeopathy, but only if a qualified homeopath is in attendance. If you have requested that a homeopath accompanies you in labour, it is wise to discuss in advance the possibility of emergency situations arising, so that your midwife and doctor are aware of your wishes before any urgent treatment is necessary.

What to expect from a visit to a homeopath
The homeopath's approach to pregnancy and childbirth is that it is a normal physiological event, and whatever treatment they offer you will merely be a means of facilitating the natural processes. At the first

visit you will be asked to tell the homeopath about your condition in your own words and without interruption – this in itself can be a part of the overall healing process, as you explain how the 'problem' for which you are seeking treatment began and think about the aspects that worry you most or cause you most discomfort. You will be asked numerous questions about your personal medical history and about this and previous pregnancies, as well as about any medical conditions which affect members of your family. Your lifestyle, diet, occupation and social activities will also be queried, as these may be relevant to the overall diagnosis and subsequent treatment. You will be asked about what makes your symptoms better or worse, whether you feel hot or cold, how the symptoms affect your mood, and so on.

A complete symptom picture is necessary in order for the homeopath to be able to prescribe the most appropriate remedy or range of remedies. Dosage is important in homeopathy – this is denoted by the number and letter after the name of the remedy on the bottle. The higher the number, the more diluted the original substance but the more powerful it becomes. The letter after the number denotes (in Roman numerals) the number of times the original substance has been diluted and succussed; thus 'X' means ten times, while 'C' means 100 times and is therefore more potent. To increase the dosage of a remedy you will need to take a tablet more frequently, *not* increase the number of tablets taken at the same time. For example, to double the dose from one tablet every four hours, you would take one tablet every two hours rather than two tablets every four hours.

Remember that if you are seeing a homeopath privately you may need to take account of the cost of the remedies suggested, on top of the consultation fees.

Precautions

As already emphasized, it is important to ensure that the correct remedy is prescribed in accordance with the precise nature of the symptoms requiring treatment. If you wish to self-administer homeopathic remedies at home, you must be careful to select the most appropriate remedy in accordance with the symptoms you are suffering at the time. After administering the first remedy, you may find that the symptoms change and the remedy will need to be adapted accordingly. If in any doubt, you should seek expert advice.

Certain substances should be avoided when you are taking homeopathic remedies because they may antidote them. These include coffee, peppermint, mint toothpastes, and substances with strong aromas such as menthol, eucalyptus, camphor and some essential oils. You should also avoid putting the tablets onto metal spoons for the same reason; it is best to tip the tablet you require into the lid of the bottle and then put it straight into your mouth. If you are giving the tablet to someone else, only they should handle it.

As a general rule, most conditions which arise in pregnancy and which you may wish to treat with homeopathy should resolve within three days of taking the remedy – if the symptoms have not changed after this time, you may have selected the incorrect remedy and should stop taking it in order to prevent a reverse proving, which could cause problems additional to the one you are already suffering.

Acupuncture

Acupuncture is a part of Traditional Chinese Medicine (TCM) and works on the principle that the body has energy lines or channels, called meridians, flowing through it from top to toe. There are 12 main meridians, each of which is connected to a major organ after which it takes its name, with additional branching meridians, totalling 365 in all. When the whole person (body, mind and spirit) is in good health, the energy (called the 'life force' or *Qi*, pronounced 'chee') flows along the meridians without interruption, but if disease or stressors affect the person, the energy flows may become blocked or too strong or too weak at certain points along one or more of the meridians – these are called acupuncture points. Inserting special, very fine acupuncture needles into the skin at these points helps to unblock them and stimulate and rebalance the energy so that it flows adequately again. Treatment can also be carried out by applying pressure to the acupuncture points – this is called 'acupressure'. The ear has a complete set of acupuncture points reflected on its surface and auricular (ear) acupuncture is a specific type of treatment.

TCM also involves the use of Chinese herbs, dietary adaptations, exercise and special massage called Tuina to aid the maintenance of health and prevention of disease. Acupuncture theory is based on an ancient Chinese text called *The Yellow Emperor's Classic of Internal Medicine*, which was compiled between 300 and 100 BC and is still considered to be the most authoritative text in the world on the subject. TCM is a normal part of mainstream healthcare in China but has only recently started to come into its own in other countries around the world.

The philosophy of TCM is very different from that of orthodox western medicine. Practitioners believe that a part can only be understood in relation to the whole, using the theory of Yin and Yang, which are two opposing forces. Yin energy implies the feminine element, with cold, darkness, internal factors, passivity and negativity, while Yang energy implies the masculine focus, with heat, light, activity, positivity and expressiveness. Ill health is a result of an imbalance between the Yin and the Yang energies which exist in us all. If an organ has too much Yin energy it will be sluggish, static and accumulate waste (for example, the gut when one is constipated); an organ which is too Yang is overactive, hot and out of control (for example, a woman experiencing hot flushes during the menopause has too much Yang energy). TCM also uses eight other principles by which all diseases and disharmonies can be described and which aid diagnosis. The aim of treatment is to rebalance the energies to facilitate harmony within the body, mind and spirit.

A great deal of research has been carried out using acupuncture, including investigating its effect on relieving pain – both in long-term illness and during labour. Various physical effects have been noticed in people receiving acupuncture, such as changes in blood pressure, heart function, the blood itself, and in the levels and functioning of hormones and other chemicals in the body. Acupuncture has been found to improve lung function in people with asthma, to ease the symptoms of stomach ulcers and to be effective in reducing hayfever.

It was once thought that the meridians were purely imaginary lines through the body, but various trials have confirmed that they do, in fact, exist: this has been shown using radio-opaque dye to map out the energy lines using X-rays, and also by measuring the output of electrical energy at the acupuncture points compared to that of the surrounding area.

Other techniques which may be used by acupuncturists or practitioners of TCM include 'cupping', in which large inverted 'cups' are placed over specific acupuncture points to draw heat from the body either to or from the area, and moxibustion (see below).

Acupuncture in pregnancy and childbirth

In TCM terms, the ability to conceive indicates that the Ren meridian is working effectively; conversely, therefore, in women suffering infertility it may be possible to stimulate the Ren channel with acupuncture so that they can become pregnant. There are, however, certain acupuncture points which should not be stimulated during pregnancy, as they may trigger uterine contractions and cause miscarriage or start labour prematurely. Labour can, in fact, be induced using acupuncture at the relevant points, and it can also be used to enhance the uterine activity when labour progress is slow.

During pregnancy, acupuncture can be immensely helpful in relieving sickness – there are numerous research trials demonstrating its effectiveness in this area. Acupuncture can also be used to treat most of the physical symptoms of pregnancy including varicose veins, skin rashes, heartburn, headaches, constipation, haemorrhoids, backache and sciatica, and sinus congestion. A specific technique called moxibustion, which involves the use of compressed herb sticks as heat sources above acupuncture points on the feet, can turn a breech baby to head-first in over 60 per cent of cases.

During childbirth, acupuncture can reduce the perception of pain from contractions, stimulate the delivery of the placenta (afterbirth) if this is delayed, and has been used in China for anaesthesia during Caesarean sections. Following the birth, acupuncture may be helpful if the mother's milk supply is slow to start, or if she is unable to pass urine or have her bowels open.

What to expect from a visit to an acupuncturist

Your acupuncturist will take a detailed history and make a visual and physical examination as appropriate in order to make a diagnosis. Fine stainless steel needles are inserted gently into the relevant acupuncture points; some sensation may be felt at the time of insertion, after which it should be relatively painless. Once the needles have been inserted they may be rotated, according to the condition being treated, and this can produce a feeling of warmth and distension around the needle which might be described as a tingling pulsation or electrical sensation. When you feel this sensation, the practitioner will know that the needle is in the correct position. The needles are usually left in place for about 20 minutes, although this can vary. Sometimes the needles are stimulated by electroacupuncture, in which light leads are attached to the handle of the needle and a mild electrical current is passed through it. The process is measured and regulated by adjusting the current and the strength and frequency of pulsations.

Precautions

Acupuncture offers an extremely effective means of dealing with many of the normal symptoms of pregnancy and birth, as well as some of the more major complications. However, it is important that you choose a practitioner who has experience of treating expectant women. All acupuncturists will be familiar with the points which should not be stimulated during pregnancy, but it is preferable that they have the additional knowledge of conventional maternity services so that communication can be ongoing.

Herbal medicine

Herbal medicine, or phytotherapy, involves the use of plant substances as medicinal products. Like other areas of complementary medicine, it is health-related rather than disease-related, with the aim of enhancing and maintaining health and well-being and focusing on inherent strengths rather than on the effects of illness and disease.

Plants are nutritional and medicinal, and are considered by herbalists and nutritional therapists to be more in harmony with the natural rhythms of the body than drugs and prescribed medicines. Various chemicals and other constituents of the plants have differing effects on the body, and when used appropriately can be very beneficial in treating a range of disorders. Usually the whole plant is used, so that all its components can work together to play their part, whereas in prescribed medicines the active ingredient has been isolated and often produced synthetically: it is this very artificiality which causes the undesirable side effects of drugs. Herbalists aim to use the lowest possible dose of the plant to achieve the therapeutic effect, which generally means that the person is able to tolerate the substance better.

The important factor here, however, is that herbs and plant medicines work in exactly the same way as manufactured drugs, and it is therefore imperative, especially in pregnancy, that the correct remedy is used. *'Natural' does not automatically mean 'safe', and there are many naturally occurring herbal remedies that are contraindicated during pregnancy.* The main difference between herbal and pharmaceutical medicines lies in the person-centred approach of the herbalist, who considers the person as a whole, rather than just looking at a set of symptoms. However, the herbalist must have a comprehensive knowledge of how the medicines affect the body, in much the same way as pharmacists and doctors are required to study the subject.

Herbal medicine has been in use for many centuries and a good proportion of today's drugs are derived from plants: for example, the contraceptive Pill originated from work which found that the wild yam has properties that can prevent pregnancy. Centuries ago, the practitioners of herbal medicine were usually women, who in the Middle Ages were often burnt at the stake on suspicion of witchcraft, simply because people did not understand what they were doing. Many women used their remedies for mothers during childbirth and for other female problems, and it was only as the more male-dominated professions of medicine and chemistry developed in the eighteenth and early nineteenth centuries that the use of herbs declined. The Industrial Revolution of the mid- and late nineteenth century also meant a population move from rural areas into more urban ones, so that the availability of land for cultivating plants was much reduced. Gradually herbal medicine disappeared, until in the late twentieth century a growing mistrust of and dissatisfaction with conventional medicine resulted in people turning once again to the more natural forms of healthcare.

Herbal medicine in pregnancy and childbirth

Many of the beneficial effects of herbs and other plants can be obtained by including the appropriate ingredients in your daily diet, although the ability of the body to absorb nutrients from food is affected by a variety of factors (see Nutritional therapy, page 61). It is also possible to self-prescribe plant foods which will have the desired action on the body, but special care should be taken during pregnancy to ensure that the correct type and dose of herbal supplements are always used.

If you are planning a pregnancy, there are many plants which can be incorporated into your diet to improve general health and increase the potential to conceive; these include chickweed, sorrel, nettles, lamb's lettuce, watercress and dandelion leaves. Such foods act as a tonic and help to improve energy, but must be eaten regularly to achieve maximum benefit.

During pregnancy, a variety of herbal remedies can be used to combat the discomforts and disorders which may occur. Pregnancy sickness, for example, may respond to peppermint or camomile tea, lemon balm or hops. Ginger is a popular remedy and is best taken as a tea made from the grated dry root, rather than as ginger biscuits which contain too much sugar. Slippery elm tablets may be available at healthfood stores and can be sucked or chewed regularly. Varicose veins, haemorrhoids and constipation can all be helped with herbal remedies: something as simple as grated raw potato applied directly to haemorrhoids can ease swelling and pain. Dandelion roots are good for constipation and lime blossom may help if you have varicose veins in the legs or vulval area. Heartburn may respond to meadowsweet, slippery elm or Iceland moss, and insomnia may be helped by camomile tea or skullcap. More major complications of pregnancy can also be treated with herbal medicine, but this should be under the supervision of a qualified practitioner; threatened miscarriage, anaemia or urinary infections can all be combated with a variety of plant substances.

Raspberry leaf is a well-known herbal remedy for assisting in the preparation of the reproductive organs for labour. The tea can be drunk from about 28 weeks of pregnancy to tone up the uterus ready for the birth, and after delivery to help the body return to the non-pregnant state. There is no real research available on raspberry leaf, but repeated reports appear to indicate its effectiveness and safety in the last 12 weeks of pregnancy, although you should avoid it if you have a history of premature labour or have previously undergone a Caesarean section.

Following delivery, there are many ways in which herbal medicine can be of use. Comfrey, marigold and lavender all assist in the healing process, especially if you have had stitches. Cabbage leaves are particularly good at relieving fluid swelling, either in the ankles in late pregnancy, or if your breasts become over-engorged as the milk supply becomes established. Research has shown that geranium (*Pelargonium*) leaves can also help regulate breast function.

What to expect from a visit to a herbalist
In order to use herbal remedies to best advantage, it is wise to consult a qualified practitioner, who will first take a history and make a diagnosis. A range of adaptations to your diet may be suggested, and it is important to realize that care is dependent on a collaborative partnership between you and your therapist: unlike consulting your family doctor, who writes out a prescription to suppress your symptoms, herbal medicine requires you to take an active part in your recovery. The herbalist may prescribe several remedies and dispense them for you there and then at the practice, or you may need to obtain them from a specialist herbal pharmacy. The remedies can be administered in a variety of ways such as an infusion or decoction (a type of tea), a tincture, or an infused oil (not to be confused with essential oils – see Aromatherapy, page 35).

Precautions

If you choose to administer herbal medicines to yourself, you need to be aware that there are some remedies which should not be taken during pregnancy; you should also be cautious with the doses. Always remember that just because these are naturally occurring plants they are not always safe to take and should be used appropriately. If you wish to purchase the herbs for your own use they should look and smell fresh, and you would be wise to buy them from a reputable supplier. Store the herbs in a dark glass jar or brown paper bag away from direct sunlight and use them within 6–12 months so that they have not degraded. Some herbs can be frozen while still fresh.

Herbs to avoid during pregnancy

Note that some of the following herbs may be used at specific times during pregnancy, but only when prescribed by a qualified herbalist.

Arbor vitae	Greater celandine	Poke root
Barberry	Juniper	Rue
Black cohosh	Marjoram	Sage
Blue cohosh	Motherwort	Squaw vine
Cinchona	Mugwort	Tansy
Golden seal	Pennyroyal	Wormwood

Aromatherapy

Aromatherapy involves the use of highly concentrated 'essential oils', extracted from various parts of different plants, for their therapeutic properties. Essential oils occur naturally in plant cells to facilitate growth and provide protection against infection and parasites, and they act in very much the same way as conventional drugs. Most of the oils smell extremely pleasant, but the term 'aromatherapy' is rather misleading because treatment does not rely only on these aromas but also on the effects of the chemicals within the oils. Different oils contain different chemicals, which have a variety of effects on both your body and your mood.

The oils are usually administered in a 'carrier oil' for massage, which in itself is very relaxing, or they may be added to the bathwater and absorbed through the skin in this way. Occasionally the oils will be prescribed for inhalation, especially if you have a cold or 'flu, but some of the oil molecules will be breathed in even when you receive them by massage for other purposes. Alternative methods of using essential oils include vaporization in a room diffuser to deodorize the air, compresses, vaginal pessaries or suppositories.

Aromatherapy has been in use for thousands of years; the ancient Egyptians, Romans and Greeks all used essential oils for a variety of medicinal purposes. In Europe, it was only at the beginning of the twentieth century that the practice began to come into its own. The term *aromatherapie* was first used in 1910 by a French chemical perfumier, René Maurice Gattefossé, who burnt his hand during an experiment and plunged it into the nearest available liquid, which happened to be essential oil of lavender. He was astounded to find that his hand healed without pain, blistering or scarring, and this led him to investigate the medicinal properties of this and other essential oils. Jean Valnet, a French doctor, used essential oils to treat soldiers in the trenches during World War I, and his books on aromatherapy are still considered to be the definitive texts in use today. Indeed, in France aromatherapy is often used by doctors of conventional medicine as an additional means of treating patients.

The oils are absorbed into the bloodstream through the skin, the mucous membranes, or the nostrils and then into the lungs. Once in the bloodstream, they behave in very much the same way as prescribed drugs, and travel around the body to specific organs where they will act, positively or negatively. They are used up in the body and any waste products are excreted via the kidneys as urine, in sweat or exhaled from the lungs. All essential oils will fight infection to a greater or lesser extent, with most being antibacterial and some able to combat fungal or viral infections. Much of the recent research has explored the potential of essential oils like tea tree to treat severe infections, such as very resistant hospital-acquired infection or the HIV virus which causes AIDS.

German researchers have undertaken several studies into the effects of the oils on mood, and have demonstrated that lavender and neroli are especially good for relaxing you and reducing blood pressure, while other oils such as jasmine and rosemary have been found to stimulate the mind and, in the case of rosemary, raise the blood pressure. This is important research, because many people believe that it is the massage alone which helps create the sense of relaxation, whereas it is now known that the chemicals in the oils facilitate this effect as well.

Aromatherapy in pregnancy and childbirth

Essential oils can be very pleasant to use at this time and you may be able to organize regular aromatherapy massages for general relaxation throughout your pregnancy. Small doses of lime, ginger or camomile oils can be effective in relieving nausea in the early weeks, and tea tree is immensely beneficial for thrush, which afflicts many expectant mothers in the later weeks. Lavender or camomile oils may help you to sleep better, and ylang ylang can be extremely relaxing if you are very stressed. Clary sage, lavender, jasmine or small doses of nutmeg can be useful for alleviating pain and discomfort in labour, and lavender may ease the pain caused by stitches after the birth.

Citrus oils can relieve constipation both before and after pregnancy and in your baby, who may also respond well to one drop of lavender on the sheet near his/her head for fretfulness or camomile for colic.

What to expect from a visit to an aromatherapist

If you choose to visit a qualified aromatherapist, you will first be asked to provide a comprehensive history to ensure that there are no existing medical conditions which could cause complications. If the aromatherapist is not also a member of your maternity care team, you should ensure that they know you are pregnant or trying to conceive so that they can take the necessary precautions.

If you are to receive a full body massage, you will be asked to undress as far as your briefs and lie on the couch. An appropriate blend of essential oils will be selected, usually in consultation with you to ensure that you like the aroma, so that the oils will be both pleasant and effective. A full body massage may take up to an hour and a half, although if you are seeking advice for a specific complaint the time may be greatly reduced. You may be given advice for self-care at home and offered more essential oils to take with you, perhaps to put in your bath.

Precautions

There are many essential oils which should not be used during pregnancy, as we do not really know enough about whether or not they are safe at this time. Some are thought to cause miscarriage or could potentially cause abnormalities in the baby if used to excess in the early weeks of pregnancy. As a general rule, it is wise to avoid most essential oils in the first three months of your pregnancy, unless they are prescribed by a qualified aromatherapist who is aware that you are pregnant. However, oils which are considered to be relatively safe to use at this time include the citrus oils such as grapefruit, orange, lime, lemon, bergamot and neroli, as well as ylang ylang, ginger and camomile in small doses.

Always try to purchase your essential oils from a reputable supplier who can vouch for their authenticity, and avoid cheap oils from market stalls or high-street supermarkets. The oils should always be contained in small, dark glass bottles to prevent the deterioration which can occur from exposure to light, oxygen and plastic. The oils should normally be diluted in a carrier oil such as sweet almond, grapeseed or avocado, but it is best to buy these separately and blend them yourself, as ready-mixed oils will deteriorate more quickly. The dose should never be more than 2 per cent (two drops of essential oil to 5ml/1 teaspoon of carrier oil) for pregnancy massage or 4 per cent (four drops to 5ml/1 teaspoon) for a bath. You should avoid using the oils neat unless you have been specifically advised to do so, as some oils contain chemicals which can irritate the skin. *Never take the oils by mouth*, as insufficient is known about the way in which the chemicals act in the digestive tract.

As mentioned above, essential oils can have a range of effects on your body and your mood, so the most appropriate oils must always be selected. A few oils can increase the effects of alcohol (although it is also wise to reduce alcohol consumption during pregnancy) and some can relax you so much that you should not immediately drive a car or operate machinery. Some essential oils are safe to use in labour but should be avoided until the baby is almost due to be born. It is known that some of the oils can interact with prescribed medicines, so you should always keep your midwife and doctor informed if you are using aromatherapy.

The most important thing you need to remember is that essential oils are not just nice-smelling perfumes: they can, if used appropriately, be highly effective in alleviating certain conditions but should always be treated with the same respect and caution that you give to prescribed pharmaceutical drugs.

Reflexology

Reflexology, or reflex zone therapy, is a system of alternative therapy based on the principle that the feet represent a map of the body and that all areas of the body are reflected on one or both feet (the hands provide a similar map but are generally less sensitive, so treatment is usually done on the feet). By working on the feet, it is theoretically possible to ease a range of discomforts or treat conditions affecting other parts of the body. Although reflexology is not technically a diagnostic technique, it is possible to identify from the feet those areas of the body which may potentially have problems, almost before they arise, or to recognize the normal changes occurring in the body at a given time. For example, I am able to identify from a woman's feet the stage of her menstrual cycle, from which ovary an egg has been released, and to estimate the date of the next menstrual period, as well as being able to predict, at the end of pregnancy, whether or not labour is imminent. It is feasible to identify which teeth require filling, areas of the body from which an organ has been removed (eg the appendix) or even to highlight major problems such as the development of a lump in the breast.

Reflexology and similar therapies evolved from ancient Chinese medicine and are thought to work on the principles of acupuncture with energy points ending in the feet, although there are various other theories about the way in which they work, including one focusing on the nerves of the body which end in the feet. Various types of foot massage appear to have been used by several ancient cultures including the Egyptians, as surmised from tomb paintings. However, it was not until the end of the nineteenth century that reflexology began to be used in the western world after an American doctor, William Fitzgerald, realized that patients often seemed instinctively to relieve pain following operations by pressing on areas of their body not directly related to the surgery. This led him to explore the concept, and he discovered that the Native American Indians applied the principle of zones throughout the body in order to treat other affected parts. He developed and refined the theory into a systematized treatment, and further work was carried out by other practitioners in America, Europe and the UK.

In reflexology, the left foot (or hand) corresponds to the left side of the body and the right foot to the right side; the top of the foot relates to the front of the body and the sole corresponds to the internal organs, with the spine zone running down the inner side of each foot. Although the procedure is very relaxing, the area being worked may also feel tender at times; the therapist uses a very precise manipulation of the feet to elicit areas which need more treatment than others. Reflexology is similar to a straightforward foot massage, although not the same, and the majority of therapists do not use oils, although some may complete a treatment with a simple foot massage with essential oils.

Reflexology in pregnancy and childbirth

Reflexology can be extremely effective for relieving specific ailments of pregnancy such as sickness, constipation, backache, headache, carpal tunnel syndrome (wrist tingling), heartburn, haemorrhoids and insomnia. Although little pregnancy-specific research has been carried out, Spanish researchers compared the effects of reflexology for headache with conventional medication and found that there was virtually no difference in their effectiveness in relieving the symptoms, but that reflexology had fewer side effects than the drugs. Similar findings were noticed in relation to constipation. General stress and anxiety can be alleviated by a course of treatment over a period of several weeks, and this may also give you the opportunity to talk through some of your fears and worries with the therapist.

During labour, reflexology may help to relieve the pain of your contractions or assist the placenta (afterbirth) to be expelled if this is delayed. Researchers in Denmark, where reflexology is frequently used alongside conventional care, have demonstrated its value in reducing contraction pain and the length of the first stage of labour in women who had a course of treatment during pregnancy and while they were in labour. Another trial by a London family doctor produced similar results.

After delivery, reflexology can be helpful for problems such as stiff neck or back following epidural anaesthetic, poor milk supply, constipation or problems with passing urine in the first few days. A course of reflexology in the early weeks of motherhood may prevent or assist in the treatment of postnatal depression. Your baby may enjoy reflexology for overall relaxation and can gain relief from colic, constipation and diarrhoea.

What to expect from a visit to a reflexologist

You will be asked to give a full history of your medical condition and lifestyle so that the therapist can build up a picture of you as a person. You will lie propped up on a couch with bare feet but will not need to undress further, unless the treatment is to be combined with another therapy. A full reflexology treatment may take up to an hour, although if you are receiving care for a specific condition the time taken may be greatly reduced; 'first aid' treatment may only take a few minutes. Usually you will be offered a course of treatment, probably three to six sessions. The practitioner will first look at your feet, as much can be learnt about your health from the shape and position of the feet and toes, the condition of the skin, and whether you have dry or hard areas or patches of redness. They will then work your feet with a relaxing technique and will identify the extent of your particular problem or your state of health; if necessary, manipulative treatment of specific zones of the feet will be carried out, which may be in the form of an intermittent or sustained pressure at precise points, depending on the findings.

After the treatment, you will be asked to rest quietly for a few moments before getting up and may be given advice on how to care for yourself before the next session. It is worth noting that your condition may worsen temporarily before it begins to get better and you may experience a response such as headache or more frequent urination as the body rids itself of toxins. You should drink plenty of water or fruit juice following the treatment to aid this process.

Precautions

If you have problems with your feet such as a verruca, this is not normally a cause for concern in relation to reflexology and may even give the practitioner further information about your condition. However, if you have major problems such as a fungal infection between your toes, severe varicose veins, a broken foot or have even lost a limb, reflexology can be performed either on the opposite foot or on your hands, because the relevant zones are the same. There are other conditions which would, however, mean that reflexology should not be performed, such as a high temperature or a serious infectious disease. Your reflexologist will need to know if you suffer from any ongoing medical conditions such as diabetes or epilepsy, or have a history of kidney or gallstones. If you have had previous miscarriages or lost a baby later in pregnancy, you should seek the advice of your midwife and doctor before receiving treatment, unless your reflexologist is also part of your conventional maternity team.

Reflexology performed appropriately will not cause problems in pregnancy, but should be used with caution if you have any pregnancy complications. If your condition is under more rigorous monitoring from your maternity carers than normal – for example, if you are expecting more than one baby, if your baby or the placenta is lying in the wrong position, or if you develop problems such as high blood pressure or bleeding – you should only receive reflexology from a practitioner who is also a midwife, doctor or maternity nurse.

Massage

Massage is the use of touch in a systematic manner in order to enhance a sense of physical and mental well-being. Massage relaxes muscles, stimulates the circulation, lowers blood pressure, helps with the excretion of waste products such as urine, faeces and sweat from the body and aids digestion. It has also been shown in many research trials to relieve pain, because touch impulses reach the brain via the nerves quicker than pain impulses, therefore blocking out some of the sensation of pain. Touch also triggers the release from the brain of endorphins and encephalins, the body's own natural pain-relieving and antidepressant chemicals, so it helps to calm and relax you, and promote the sense of well-being.

There are many different types of massage practised all over the world; some are gentle and relaxing, others work more deeply and are more vigorous. Massage is not difficult to learn and your partner could be shown a few simple techniques to help you in labour. The most pleasant aspect of massage is the fact that it is a 'nurturing' touch rather than just a 'functional' touch – in the western world, in particular, we are usually keen to maintain our own personal space and this results, in some cultures, in people rarely touching each other except in intimate relationships. Unfortunately, in some countries massage has gained a reputation as being merely a beauty therapy for pampering people (usually seen to be 'rich women'), or as something rather sleazy with a sexual connotation that is only slowly being discarded.

Massage usually requires the practitioner to use an oil or other substance to help the hands to glide over the surface of the skin and so prevent the friction of skin-to-skin contact. This may be a base massage oil such as sweet almond, grapeseed, avocado, sunflower, safflower or apricot or peach kernel, or talcum powder – or soap and water will suffice if nothing else is available. Often essential oils (see Aromatherapy, page 35) are added to the base oil for specific therapeutic purposes, although aromatherapy is a separate therapy in its own right.

Massage in pregnancy and labour

Regular massage during pregnancy can be relaxing for both you and your baby. Pregnancy is a time of myriad worries and concerns and can be exhausting, especially if you are continuing to work. Massage provides a short period of 'time out' for yourself. It can also be effective in relieving some of the aches and pains of pregnancy and in reducing the impact of 'baby blues' or preventing depression.

Gentle abdominal massage, performed in a clockwise direction, can stimulate excretory processes and so relieve the constipation which many women suffer at this time. Backache that is a result of hormonal and postural changes can be eased by massage to the lower back, and swollen ankles can be reduced, albeit temporarily, by upwards massage of the legs. Head massage is wonderful both for relaxation and for the sometimes unbearable, but normal, headaches of early pregnancy.

You may be fortunate enough to find antenatal classes in your area which focus on teaching you and your partner or intended birth companion how to use massage techniques for labour. Back, lower abdomen, shoulder and neck massage are all pleasant, relaxing and partially pain-relieving when you are in labour. Foot massage is also good, because women in labour quite literally get 'cold feet' as blood is directed to those parts of the body that are working hardest.

Some women like to undertake massage of the perineum (the area between the vagina and anus) in the last few weeks of pregnancy and during labour to help stretch the area and reduce the likelihood of having an episiotomy (a cut to enlarge the birth opening) and stitches. Massage of the clitoris is also carried out by some women in an attempt to start labour if they are overdue. Nipple massage during labour can accelerate the output of the hormone responsible for uterine contractions, so may help if labour is slow or if the placenta (afterbirth) is slow to separate.

Baby massage

Gentle systematic touching and stroking of your baby is one of the most wonderful acts you can perform for him/her. Baby massage has become very popular and there are many classes available to teach you how to do this. It helps to relax your baby and promote the development of the relationship between the two of you. You will probably experience a sense of calmness as well while you are doing the massage for your baby.

Massage of the baby's tummy can alleviate colic and constipation, and general body massage will aid the onset of sleep and calm your baby if s/he is fractious. A lot of research has been undertaken, primarily in the USA, on the short- and long-term effects of baby massage, and has found that regular massage can increase the levels of beneficial chemicals in the baby's blood, which improves the prognosis for babies born very prematurely and increases their long-term intellectual prospects.

What to expect from a visit to a massage therapist

You will be asked to tell the therapist about your medical history and lifestyle, and the reasons why you have chosen to consult them. A plan of treatment will be discussed with you if you are to have several sessions, although you may simply have decided to receive one massage at a particular time for relaxation. However, if you have not had a massage before, the degree of relaxation may not be as deep after only one treatment as it would be after several because the effects are cumulative.

If you are to receive a full body massage, you will be asked to undress down to your underwear and lie on the couch; you will then be covered with towels, both for your dignity and because your body temperature may drop slightly while you are having the massage. You should be offered the opportunity to visit the toilet before you start so that your bladder is empty: feeling the need to urinate half-way through the massage is not only uncomfortable but will hinder your ability to relax! If the therapist has come to your home, you should ensure that you will not be disturbed by the telephone or other people entering the room, and you may wish to dim the lights. Some massage therapists offer you a choice of soft music to assist in the relaxation process. You will be asked to remove jewellery, watch, hair ornaments and possibly make-up if your face is to be massaged.

The massage will probably commence on your back and proceed down the backs of your legs, before you are asked to turn over so that the massage can be completed. Different therapists work in different orders, but a full body massage will include the fronts of your legs, arms, chest, abdomen, and face and head. If you do not wish any part of your body to be massaged and/or exposed, you need to discuss this with the therapist before they commence. This applies particularly to the breast area, about which you may feel uncomfortable, either physically or mentally, especially towards the end of your pregnancy when you may already be producing the colostrum, or pre-milk, for the baby.

Following the massage, you will be given a short while to 'come round' and may be offered a drink. You should be given advice to drink plenty of water over the next few hours and other information for self-care may be offered.

Precautions

You will need to ensure that the therapist you choose to visit is experienced in treating pregnant women. They should be aware that massage to your lower back is probably best avoided during the first three months and should take care to note any pregnancy complications you may have. You should also check whether or not they intend to use essential oils and if so ensure that they are a fully qualified aromatherapist as well as masseuse (see Aromatherapy – Precautions, page 38).

Care should be taken to help you find the most comfortable position for the massage: you may feel comfortable lying on your front to receive back massage early in pregnancy, but will not do so later and should be offered alternatives such as sitting upright and leaning forwards against a support. Also, in late pregnancy you should be advised not to lie flat on your back for too long, as the weight of your baby presses on the blood vessels which return blood to your heart and can cause you to feel dizzy and faint due to a drop in blood pressure, and may also temporarily slow down the oxygen supply to your baby. You should therefore lie slightly propped up on two or three pillows.

If you wish to learn how to perform massage for your baby, you should contact a registered instructor of infant massage. It is best to refrain from taking your baby to the session if s/he is at all unwell, although fractiousness as a result of teething discomfort may be eased by a good relaxing massage.

Shiatsu

Shiatsu, from a Japanese word meaning 'finger pressure', evolved from an earlier form of Japanese massage called Anma (or Tuina in China – see Acupuncture, page 29). Although the principles have been used since the sixth century, shiatsu is a twentieth-century system of medicine incorporating the newer western knowledge of anatomy, physiology and physiotherapy techniques, and was formally recognized in Japan in 1964.

Shiatsu uses simple pressure and holding techniques with gentle stretching while the client remains clothed. It is based on Traditional Chinese Medicine (TCM) and, like acupuncture, uses the principles of meridians, or energy lines, throughout the body. In shiatsu, however, rather than the needles of acupuncture the practitioner applies pressure with their thumbs, fingers, elbows and even knees to the relevant points along the meridians to balance the body's life force, or *Ki* in Japanese.

Investigations by two Japanese researchers seemed to indicate that the meridians lie in the tissues of the body that connect different parts to one another and in the membranous covering of organs and muscles. They surmised that these tissues act as conductors of electrical energies within the body from one part to another and that this is, in fact, the meridian network used in TCM. Shiatsu massage is thought to induce small electrical currents that will be conducted away from the point of pressure and act on distant parts of the body. In research trials, these electrical currents have been found to increase the amount of oxygen in the tissues and improve the circulation, as well as aiding the excretion of toxins and waste products from the body. Shiatsu massage also helps to regulate nerve function, to strengthen resistance to disease, and to make the joints more flexible.

Shiatsu in pregnancy and childbirth

Shiatsu is a 'hands-on' therapy and therefore in itself can be reassuring and relaxing. Oriental medicine considers pregnancy to be one of the focal points of a woman's life, one of the 'Gateways of Change' which occur at times of great hormonal upheaval, and a period when care should be taken with your health. Shiatsu can assist in strengthening your energy levels to help you cope with the fluctuations in your physical and emotional state. The relaxation which can be obtained from shiatsu is important for both you and your baby, particularly as the Japanese believe that the time spent in the uterus, before birth, determines one-third of an individual's ultimate physical, mental and social functioning.

On a physical level, shiatsu can relieve tiredness and fatigue and trigger the flow of endorphins, the body's natural 'feel-good factor', and is thought to stimulate energy levels along the Kidney meridian, which often becomes depleted during pregnancy. Oriental medicine attributes problems in pregnancy such as low backache, swollen ankles, breathlessness, chronic coughs, insomnia, and vaginal and urinary infections to a depletion of Kidney energy – energy which runs along the meridian that passes through the kidney but also affects other organs. Other meridians which may suffer low energy levels at this time include the Spleen and Stomach meridians, which may result in constipation, leg cramps, haemorrhoids, heartburn, nausea and poor milk supply. It is therefore possible, in TCM terms, to treat all these complaints with shiatsu.

During labour, shiatsu massage can help with relieving pain, discomfort and exhaustion, and may stimulate more effective uterine contractions if labour is slow to start or the rate of progress is slow. It will also help if the placenta is retained for any length of time following the birth of the baby. Afterwards, shiatsu can increase milk production, help to prevent (or prevent worsening of) postnatal depression and ease constipation.

Shiatsu massage for the baby is very relaxing for both mother and child, and uses a combination of Swedish massage techniques and shiatsu with oil on the baby's skin. It can also treat specific conditions such as colic, vomiting, constipation, diarrhoea and sleeplessness.

Later on in the first year of your baby's life, shiatsu may help in the treatment of poor appetite, excess catarrh, coughs, earache and teething troubles.

What to expect from a visit to a shiatsu practitioner

A full case history will be taken prior to any treatment and a diagnosis made in terms of TCM theory. There are several different forms of diagnosis. Many practitioners concentrate on palpation of the abdomen ('hara') in order to assess the relative energy in each of the internal organs; others will measure the frequency and strength of numerous pulses around the body. The tongue is also used to assess the state of your health.

If you are to receive a full shiatsu massage for relaxation and general toning of the energy levels, you will be asked to lie on a mat on the floor fully clothed (it is best to wear loose clothing such as T-shirt and leggings). The practitioner will then work systematically around your body, applying pressure to all the shiatsu points to tone, sedate or move the energies. Specific emphasis may be put on some points which warrant more in-depth treatment. This may feel like a 'good hurt', a dull aching, bruised sensation, or it can at times be painful. However, as the energy is dissipated by the pressure, the pain should lessen. If you have requested treatment for a specific complaint, you may sit on a chair, perhaps with your feet up on a stool, and pressure will be applied to the appropriate points.

Precautions

There are certain points which, as in acupuncture, are contraindicated during pregnancy as they may initiate labour contractions, including some on the hands and shoulders, and particularly the area of the lower inner leg and the lower back and sacrum. A therapist may decline to treat you if you are suffering any active skin or infectious diseases, slipped discs in your back, varicose veins or have a history of thrombosis. You should also discontinue treatment if complications arise in pregnancy which require the attention of your obstetrician.

Hypnotherapy

Hypnotherapy, or hypnosis, is usually described as the process of inducing a state of deep physical and mental relaxation, with altered consciousness, similar to the daydreaming state, which enables the subconscious mind to be accessed in order to help the client make changes in their habits or behaviour. Hypnosis is not a means of making people do things they do not wish to do, because the process requires a degree of partnership between the client and the therapist in order for it to empower the client to take responsibility for their own actions.

Hypnosis has often been quoted as an effective therapy for helping people to stop smoking or lose weight, and indeed it can be very successful, but the client must be sufficiently motivated to change their behaviour. On the other hand, it can be very helpful for people with phobias, such as fear of visiting the dentist, or in order to break bedwetting habits in (older) children.

Hypnotherapy in pregnancy and childbirth

Hypnotherapy can be a very valuable tool if you are especially stressed during pregnancy, and can offer you a way of inducing a relaxed state by means of a 'post-hypnotic suggestion': a visual, physical or mental trigger which you use to relax yourself. This is particularly good for women who have previously had a traumatic pregnancy or labour, or who have lost a baby. You can also be taught relaxation techniques if you have fears or concerns regarding specialized examinations such as amniocentesis or internal examinations.

Research has shown that hypnotherapy can help to relieve some of the physical symptoms of pregnancy such as allergic itching or eczema, sickness, constipation or insomnia. Women who suffer such severe sickness that they require hospital admission have responded well to hypnotherapy, because there are often emotional factors which make the sickness worse than normal.

There is some evidence to suggest that hypnosis may also assist in relaxing mothers sufficiently to turn breech babies to head-first, and a small trial demonstrated that it may be effective in prolonging the subsequent pregnancies of women who had suffered previous premature labours.

It is, however, in the control of pain perception during labour that hypnotherapy comes into its own. Some large research trials have found very positive results in easing the pain and discomfort of labour, and hypnotherapy may also reduce the length of labour. The need for conventional pain-relieving drugs is usually reduced, with lower doses required, in women who have also had hypnotherapy, and the after-effects of the drugs are also greatly reduced. There is some evidence to suggest that the condition of the baby at birth may be better in women who have received hypnotherapy, although this may simply be due to the reduction in the amount of pain medication. Anxiety regarding planned Caesarean section may also be eased by a course of hypnosis.

What to expect from a visit to a hypnotherapist

A comprehensive history will be taken and you will be encouraged to talk about the way you feel in relation to your particular reason for consulting the hypnotherapist. You will then be asked to make yourself comfortable, either in a chair or perhaps lying on a couch, and probably to close your eyes.

The therapist will then talk to you quietly and take you through a series of images in your mind, which can later be used as trigger thoughts to help your condition. This may take up to an hour but will vary according to your condition and the individual therapist. At the end of the session you will be asked to 'come round' slowly and to open your eyes at a given cue. You will feel relaxed and perhaps sleepy when you are roused, but should soon feel able to get up.

Precautions

Unfortunately, popular television shows have done little to enhance the credibility or respectability of hypnotherapy. Occasionally the inappropriate use of entertainment hypnosis results in traumatic effects for an individual, which may lead to a court case and be reported in the media. It must be emphasized that it is not the hypnosis itself that causes long-term psychological problems, but the way in which it is used. Entertainment hypnosis takes no account of the person's medical history or psychological state, nor of the ridicule and humiliation which can result from being induced to act in a way that is humorous, for the benefit of the audience. This can damage the person's self-image and lead to feelings of insecurity, depression and distrust of others.

It is therefore essential that you only consult a hypnotherapist who is registered with a national regulatory organization. Many hypnotherapists are also psychotherapists, some are doctors, and recommendation by word of mouth is often one of the better means of finding a reputable therapist. Your therapist should take a careful history to ensure that any imagery they intend to use is not going to be detrimental to your health; for example, it would be inappropriate to use the image of rivers and waterfalls with someone who has previously suffered a near-drowning experience. *The one absolute contraindication to hypnotherapy treatment is if you have a personal history of psychosis or other serious mental disorder.*

Bach flower remedies

Bach (pronounced 'batch') flower remedies belong to the group of complementary therapies known as 'vibrational' or energy medicine, as does homeopathy – in other words, they do not work in the same way as conventional drugs and it is difficult to explain exactly how they do work.

Dr Edward Bach was a doctor and homeopath at the beginning of the twentieth century who, through his research, found that certain plant substances, when used in homeopathic dilutions, appeared to have a subtle energy which gave them the ability to treat not the physical but the emotional aspects of disease and disorder. The remedies are not prepared in the same way as homeopathic medicines, by dilution and succussion (see Homeopathy, page 24); instead, the petals of the flowers are exposed to sunlight while in water, and then preserved in an equal amount of brandy: this mix is called the mother tincture. Another method is to boil the petals in spring water for half an hour, then strain the liquid and dilute it with an equal amount of brandy.

There are 38 remedies in the range developed by Dr Bach, plus a composite Rescue Remedy. (Other ranges of flower remedies using different plants are also available in many countries, but these are not discussed here.)

The Bach flower remedies

Agrimony for people who hide their true feelings behind a cheerful face
Aspen for fear of the unknown
Beech for perfectionists, who are intolerant and critical
Centaury for those who find it difficult to say 'no', who are exploited
Cerrato for indecision, constantly seeking reassurance, ditherers
Cherry plum for rage, fear of losing control
Chestnut bud for those who do not learn from past experiences or mistakes
Clematis for absent-mindedness, inattentiveness, those who are easily bored
Crab apple for poor body image, self-disgust, sense of uncleanliness
Elm for feeling overwhelmed by responsibility
Gentian for depression, despondency, pessimism
Gorse for despair
Heather for self-centredness, self-obsession
Holly for jealousy, hatred, paranoia, suspicion
Honeysuckle for nostalgia, living in the past
Hornbeam for emotional weariness, 'Monday morning feeling'
Impatiens for impatience, irritability
Larch for lack of self-confidence, fear of failure
Mimulus for fear of known things
Mustard for depression of unknown origin
Oak for stalwarts, temporarily overwhelmed by exhaustion
Olive for physical or mental tiredness
Pine for guilt, remorse, self-blame
Red chestnut for over-concern for others, fearing impending disaster

Rock rose for terror and panic
Rock water for the perfectionist, who is strong willed
Scleranthus for inability to make decisions
Star of Bethlehem for shock, bereavement and trauma
Sweet chestnut for complete despair and unbearable unhappiness
Vervain for those who have pushed themselves too far
Vine for ambitious, autocratic, dominant personalities
Walnut for protection from change and outside influences
Water violet for reserved, reclusive, isolated people
White chestnut for unwanted worries and thoughts, inability to concentrate
Wild oat for those needing a change of direction, at a crossroads
Wild rose for those without ambition or direction in life
Willow for self-pity, resentment, bitterness

Rescue Remedy is a combination of five of the 38 remedies: rock rose, Star of Bethlehem, impatiens, cherry plum and clematis. This is a wonderful anti-stress remedy, good for nerves, panic, anxiety and hysteria. It is a useful remedy to keep with you at all times and could be used if you dislike having blood taken at your antenatal clinic, or feel stressed before an internal examination. If you are to undergo special tests, investigations or procedures, it may help to ease the tense, slightly panicky feelings you may have – for example, before an amniocentesis, or when your labour is being induced or you are to have a planned Caesarean section. A cream version of Rescue Remedy is also available, which contains crab apple as an extra ingredient for its cleansing properties.

Bach flower remedies in pregnancy and childbirth

It is difficult to detail precisely what you should take for relief of emotional feelings in pregnancy because only you will know what you are feeling. Bach flower remedies can quite easily be self-prescribed with the aid of the leaflets available at the point of purchase, although treatment may be more effective through consulting a registered practitioner, who will usually be offering the remedies in conjunction with another therapy.

Walnut is a particularly good remedy at this time to protect you from the huge changes that both your body and your lifestyle are undergoing. Mimulus can be effective if you have vague worries about the impending birth but are not sure what it is that you are worrying about, whereas larch will calm you if you know what you are concerned about. Scleranthus may be helpful if you have to make a decision, perhaps about whether or not to give up work, or about whether you should have an invasive investigation such as an amniocentesis. If you experience recurrent negative thoughts or if you are having a lot of vivid dreams you could try white chestnut, and if you feel overwhelmed by the responsibility of having a baby, elm may help. If you are weary and tired, especially in labour, olive can be an effective remedy.

Rescue Remedy is invaluable in a glass of water during labour to relieve the tension and anxiety, most particularly towards the end of the first stage, just before the baby is ready to be born. If problems arise in labour which were unexpected and you are unable to follow your anticipated plan for the birth, you may find gentian helpful. Crab apple may ease the feeling of uncleanliness which you may have after the birth when you are still discharging blood. Later, when your baby is very demanding you could try gorse if you feel at the end of your tether and in complete despair. If you are struggling on even when you are very exhausted, oak can help.

When using the main range of 38 remedies, you should select those most appropriate to your symptoms and use two drops of each in spring water three times daily until your emotions change. If you are using the Rescue Remedy, you should take four drops either neat on your tongue or in a small glass of water. In an emergency it can also be dabbed onto your temples or inner wrists and will be absorbed through the skin.

Precautions

Although these remedies are preserved in brandy they are, as far as is known, safe to take during pregnancy, so unless you have any moral objections to the alcohol content, you should not worry as you are literally taking only a few drops at a time. There is no real research available on how the remedies actually work, although one or two studies have been carried out on the Rescue Remedy to demonstrate its effectiveness.

Alexander technique

The Alexander technique has been in use for over a hundred years and was originally devised by and named after an Australian actor called Frederick Alexander. He suffered from continual throat problems, especially prior to going on stage, and discovered that when he was nervous, his neck, back and head became tense, causing a tightening of the jaw and shoulder muscles and leading to a loss of voice together with neck and throat problems. Alexander taught himself to alter his posture and to recognize when the muscles were tense so that he could acquire better control over his voice and his body. He began to help fellow actors to increase their awareness of the alignment of their bodies and gradually trained others in his methods. He also made links between the physical and mental aspects of the individual and realized that it was not possible to separate them.

The Alexander technique is now used to teach people how to eliminate the bad habits of body misuse, including muscle tension and poor breathing techniques, which may have triggered physical or emotional disorders. Movement and posture is mainly habitual and we learn an action by repetition until we no longer need to think consciously about how to do it – for example, learning to drive a car. During childhood we learn physical skills by copying and practice, and we also observe attitudes and responses to situations such as anxiety or anger. It is therefore possible that we learn poor movement, co-ordination and posture in our early lives, but this may be made worse by developing bad habits following trauma or illness, or by seeking to hide and protect those parts of ourselves with which we are dissatisfied. An example of this might be the adolescent who has grown very tall much more quickly than friends of the same age and who consequently slouches in an attempt not to stand out from the crowd. Unfortunately, this slouching posture becomes a habit that is difficult to break, even when it is no longer necessary, and may eventually lead to problems such as neck curvature, headaches and lower back pain.

Alexander technique in pregnancy and childbirth

Pregnancy can be an extremely stressful time, both physically and emotionally. The increase in your weight coupled with the influence of pregnancy hormones on the muscles, ligaments and joints leads to changes in your posture which can result in backache, headaches and other problems. Although it is best if you have learnt the Alexander technique before you become pregnant, so that you will already have learnt good postural habits to help you avoid some of the aches and pains of pregnancy, you can still use it effectively by attending sessions at this time.

The Alexander teacher assists you to become aware of how your body is functioning and to recognize muscular tensions so that you can make an effort to relax them. Breathing techniques are taught which not only help you during the pregnancy but are particularly useful when you are in labour. Pelvic floor exercises may also be encouraged, as well as abdominal muscle relaxation, which aid good general health but are also specific to pregnancy and childbirth. Advice is given about more efficient ways to use your body when standing, walking, sitting, lifting or carrying during pregnancy or in the early days of parenthood.

Squatting is encouraged as a means of opening up the pelvis most effectively for the birth of your baby, although many women find this immensely tiring unless they are accustomed to it, so it is probably best kept for the second stage of labour when the baby is actually being born. After the birth, the Alexander technique can help you maintain a good posture for breastfeeding your baby as well as assist you in re-adapting to the non-pregnant posture.

What to expect from a visit to an Alexander teacher

The focus of the sessions you have with an Alexander teacher is not so much on providing a treatment as on teaching you, usually on a one-to-one basis, about the way your body works and how you can help yourself to make it work more efficiently, by making adaptations to the ways in which you move and hold yourself. The sessions are suitable for people with virtually any physical condition, especially pregnant women.

The lessons are gentle and non-threatening, and you will not have to undress; although the teacher may need to touch you to help you correct your posture, the touch should not be intrusive. Most lessons last about half an hour and the number and frequency of future lessons will be discussed with you. The teacher's aim is to increase your awareness of co-ordination and movement on the principle of the relationship between your head, neck and back, and you are very much a partner in the process.

Precautions

You need to make sure that your teacher is fully qualified and is aware that you are pregnant. Otherwise, there are no real precautions to consider, although if you are asked to do something which feels too uncomfortable you should inform the teacher.

Hydrotherapy

Hydrotherapy involves the use of water as a means of treatment. This includes swimming and exercises in water, where the buoyancy and weightlessness help movement and flexibility and encourage aerobic exercise. Hydrotherapy also includes other methods of using water therapeutically, such as floatation tanks or the internal use of water such as colonic irrigation, but these are not covered in this book as they are inappropriate for pregnant women.

Hydrotherapy in pregnancy and childbirth

Exercising in water will help you to maintain fitness and muscle function and to improve circulation during pregnancy. If you are considering being in water during labour, antenatal classes will accustom you to the sensation of floating. Breathing techniques are also included, which are helpful in preparation for labour. The combination of practising the exercises and the tension created around you by the water can be useful in alleviating backache or the pain of throbbing varicose veins. Some research appears to indicate that water exercises during pregnancy increase the flow of blood to the uterus and also help to reduce fluid retention such as swollen ankles. Even your baby may benefit if you choose to exercise in water rather than in normal 'land-based' classes, because in water your temperature-regulating mechanism will cause fewer changes to the baby's heartbeat.

After the birth, you may be able to continue attending the classes to assist you to lose weight.

What to expect from an exercise-in-water class

You may find exercise-in-water classes offered specifically for expectant mothers to attend in later pregnancy, both as a way of exercising and preparing for labour and in order to meet other mothers-to-be. Often music is used to help you co-ordinate the simple exercises as they are taught by your instructor, and even if you are unable to swim you will find the sessions beneficial: usually they are carried out in the shallow end of the pool.

Precautions

You should ensure that any classes you attend during pregnancy are conducted by properly qualified teachers who are experienced in teaching both swimming and pregnant women. Any reputable class will ensure that there are lifesavers present, and you may also find that a midwife or other professional from the conventional maternity services is on hand to give advice and answer questions. If you have any complications during your pregnancy you should inform the teacher, and if you think that your bag of waters may have broken and that you could be starting labour you should not attend. The temperature of the pool should be warm but not too hot and your own temperature should not exceed 39°C – if you begin to feel overheated, you should get out of the pool.

Water birth

It may be possible to arrange for you to labour in a birthing pool and even for the baby to be born in the water, whether this is at home or in a maternity unit. However, this will require careful planning and preparation, so you need to make a decision about it fairly early in your pregnancy. Some maternity units may be able to offer you a water birth service as one of their standard options, but many will need to make special arrangements. In this case, or if you plan to have your baby at home, the responsibility for preparations – including hire and assembly of the specially constructed pool – will generally be yours.

Research has shown that labour pain is generally reduced considerably in women who choose to labour in water and that it encourages a greater depth of relaxation. This in turn facilitates a more satisfactory outcome to birth, especially as you are likely to adopt the most favourable position for delivery: this reduces damage to your pelvic floor and permits a more gentle introduction to the world for your baby.

Precautions

If you are choosing to have your baby at home, you should ensure that the pool you hire is designated specially for childbirth and you must check the strength of the floors in your home before filling the pool with water. A full birthing pool weighs in the region of 500kg, which may be too heavy for some floors, particularly if you live in a flat or apartment. You may also need to provide an additional source of water, as the domestic water tank may not hold enough to fill the pool.

If your condition remains stable and within normal parameters during pregnancy, there is no reason why you should not achieve a water birth if that continues to be your choice. However, if any changes take place which indicate that possible complications may occur you should be guided by your midwife as to whether it remains safe for you to labour, or continue to labour, in the pool. You will probably be asked to get out of the pool once the baby has been born in order to deliver the placenta (afterbirth), because this is the time when some mothers can bleed profusely and it is safer to deal with this when you are 'on land'.

Nutritional therapy

Nutritional therapy involves the use of dietary measures to ensure health and well-being. It focuses not only on the amount and quality of the food you eat but also on the way in which it is absorbed into the body and used. A vast range of factors affect our ability to absorb and utilize nutrients from food: these include lifestyle, environmental pollution, any medication we may be taking, our age, gender and general health. It is possible to visit a practitioner who specializes in nutritional therapy, although many other complementary practitioners will incorporate it into their advice to clients.

Nutritional therapy in pregnancy and childbirth

Good nutrition is vital to help you conceive and successfully carry your baby until s/he is developed and grown enough to be born safely. Pregnancy makes major demands on your body – and the baby will take what s/he needs first, so if you are undernourished it is you who will suffer.

Although you may be given dietary advice by your maternity professionals, nutritional therapy goes one step further and looks in detail at your health in relation to the food you are (or are not) eating. For example, you may have been eating a very well-balanced diet but have been on the contraceptive Pill before you became pregnant. The Pill has been shown by research to interfere with the body's ability to absorb zinc and vitamin B6 from the food you eat, so it may cause problems with actually getting pregnant or, if you do conceive, can increase the likelihood and severity of pregnancy sickness. Treatment would include increasing the amount of foods which contain zinc and B6, as well as using vitamin and mineral supplements to reverse the deficiency. Another example is the effect of drinking vast amounts of tea. This increases the chances of constipation because tannin in the tea slows down the movement of the gut; tea also interferes with absorption of vitamin C through the stomach wall and this in turn can influence your body's ability to absorb iron from the food you eat – so you are more likely to become anaemic in pregnancy.

Precautions

While it is possible to read books on how to use your diet more effectively to enhance your health, it must be stressed that you should *not* take to extremes any of the suggestions you may find. A varied, well-balanced diet is the best way to ensure that you are receiving a range of nutrients: going 'overboard' to increase one type of nutrient may be harmful, because it may suppress the levels of other nutrients in your body and so lead to other problems. It is best if you make any adaptations to your diet under expert supervision and be guided throughout by your conventional maternity professionals.

Relaxation techniques

There are many complementary techniques which will aid relaxation – several of those already discussed are invaluable in helping you to stay calm and will reduce the effects of stress and anxiety. This section briefly describes some of the methods by which you can achieve relaxation.

Exercise in pregnancy

Exercise is well documented as a means of reducing stress and, of course, maintaining fitness. It stimulates the body's own anti-stress chemicals – endorphins and encephalins – from the brain, aids circulation, and improves heart and lung function. During pregnancy exercise can be very effective in helping to reduce the impact of some of the physical symptoms, but care must be taken as to how vigorous the exercise becomes. Certain sports are considered unsafe during pregnancy – these include scuba diving, contact sports such as football and rugby, weightlifting, competitive events, saunas, jacuzzis and whirlpools, and dangerous sports such as parachuting, rock climbing, pot-holing or bungie jumping.

Other sports may be relatively safe but can become unsafe as your pregnancy progresses; these should only be continued with caution after discussion with your instructors and your doctor, midwife or maternity nurse. Such sports include horse-riding, gymnastics, weight training, skiing (downhill or water), racket sports, netball, running, golf and any sports involving balance.

Those activities which can be continued throughout pregnancy, so long as you are sensible and do not over-exert yourself, include swimming, cycling, walking and gentle jogging, aerobics, yoga and Tai Chi (see below and page 65).

Precautions

You should ensure that your instructor is aware that you are pregnant. You must wear good supportive footwear to provide a cushioning against impact, and a well-fitting maternity bra, including under a swimsuit. Make sure that you warm up and cool down gradually as directed by your instructor, and that you sip plenty of water throughout the exercise period and afterwards. You should work at a level where you are slightly out of breath but still able to carry on a conversation; your pulse rate should not exceed 140 beats a minute. If you begin to feel unwell you should decrease your activity gradually and then seek advice from your instructor, family doctor or midwife.

Yoga

Yoga is a movement therapy that is usually combined with meditation in order to harmonize the well-being of body, mind and spirit, which in turn leads to good health. Yoga exercise improves posture, flexibility, muscle tone and breathing, which benefits the circulation and the body's intake and use of oxygen from the air we breathe. Waste products are also excreted from the body more rapidly, and the nervous and hormonal systems function better.

Yoga in pregnancy and childbirth

Yoga is very suitable for pregnant women because its focus is on achieving and maintaining optimum physical and mental well-being.

The physical postures which can be adapted for pregnancy and then learnt will encourage strength and suppleness, while the gentle stretching exercises will maintain free movement and help to improve posture. Backache can be relieved by adopting yoga positions, as can some of the other symptoms of pregnancy such as constipation. As with the Alexander technique (see page 56), yoga breathing exercises aid relaxation during pregnancy and can be of enormous help when you are in labour. Learning to meditate can assist you in coping with some of the stresses of being pregnant and will increase your sense of being in control.

What to expect from a yoga class

In beginner classes, simple postures, or 'asanas', are taught and assumed slowly and gently without straining. Each asana is maintained for a few minutes and then gently released, followed by a short period of relaxation before assuming the next position. Concentration is very important, as is breathing slowly, regularly and deeply in co-ordination with the type of asana being used. Initially, some of the asanas can be uncomfortable until you are more familiar with them and your joints loosen up.

There may be a variety of yoga classes available in your area, but you need to ensure that the philosophy of the one you choose is in keeping with your own views on life. Some classes are very much focused on the physical improvements which can be achieved through the exercises, while others include much more meditation and emphasize the eastern philosophy from which yoga is derived. Others may include aspects of both extremes. It may be possible to find classes which are specific to pregnancy, although non-specific classes may welcome you as well.

Precautions

It is important that the yoga teacher knows you are pregnant, especially if you attend a class which also has non-pregnant people in it, as some of the exercises and postures must be adapted for you. There is no danger in practising yoga so long as you are careful and avoid postures which over-stretch your pelvic ligaments.

Tai Chi

Tai Chi is a gentle form of exercise based on an ancient Chinese martial art. It is usually taught in classes and can be practised at home. The movements are very slow and flow smoothly in a prescribed sequence. Tai Chi exercises every part of the body yet helps to conserve energy because none of the movements is superfluous. There are 108 basic movements, usually taught in one of two sequences. You are unlikely to feel tired after a session – in fact, you should feel rejuvenated; Tai Chi is suitable for you however fit or unfit you may be. Tai Chi is especially beneficial for people with heart problems, high blood pressure and conditions where movement is impaired. Research has shown that it can be physically, mentally and socially advantageous for older women after the menopause.

Tai Chi in pregnancy and childbirth

Attending Tai Chi classes or practising at home during pregnancy will help to maintain your health and sense of well-being, reduce feelings of stress, reduce blood pressure if it is raised, and may help with relieving backache, sciatica, leg cramps, swollen ankles and other discomforts. Mentally, it may assist in preparing you for the rigours of labour and the birth, and for your changing role in becoming a mother.

What to expect from a Tai Chi class

Specialist classes for expectant mothers will ensure that the whole class is geared to your specific needs and will also give you an opportunity to meet other mothers-to-be. Some of the movements will be adapted to ensure that they are suitable for pregnant women, and those which involve an element of 'bearing down' will not be practised.

Precautions

It is safe to perform Tai Chi movements from 24 to 34 weeks of pregnancy. There are no other real precautions, but it is best to inform your teacher that you are pregnant.

A simple relaxation technique

This relaxation technique can be used whenever you feel tense or anxious, not only in labour but also during pregnancy, such as when you are having blood taken or undergoing an internal examination. Your partner can use it, too, and may find it useful for relieving tension while he is with you during labour.

Imagine what happens when you are very stressed – you clench your fists and your jaw, hunch your shoulders and press your thighs together. Your breathing becomes short and shallow and you may even hold your breath, literally forgetting to breathe. Relaxation consists of being able to regulate your breathing to avoid hyperventilating when you are stressed; in addition, your body needs to recognize the difference between muscles which are tense, those which are extended and those which are relaxed.

In order to be in control of your breathing, start by audibly forcing your breath out of your lungs through your mouth – this is similar to a sigh of relief. Then, at your own pace and depth, concentrate on breathing out slowly (Sigh Out Slowly = SOS) and let breathing in take care of itself. If you focus on the exhalation, you will prevent the hyperventilation or rapid shallow breathing which occurs when your breath literally 'runs away with you'. It is natural to try to hold your breath and forget to breathe again, so by emptying your lungs as much as possible you will be stimulated to inhale air and continue breathing deeply and regularly.

Now, so that you can recognize muscle relaxation, try clenching your fist as tightly as you can: the muscles in your hand are contracted. Now stretch your hand so that your fingers are straight and taut: the muscles are extended. Now stop stretching your hand and let it just rest on your lap: your hand muscles are neither contracted nor extended – they are relaxed.

The complete exercise given here involves the processes of extension and relaxation for each group of muscles throughout your body. Start working through the exercise slowly, but practise regularly during your pregnancy so that, by the time you go into labour, you can induce the feeling of relaxation almost in one single action. You may find it easier to have someone read the instructions aloud to you.

- Settle yourself in a comfortable position, either sitting or lying well supported by cushions.
- Concentrate on your breathing (in labour, as a contraction is beginning), as explained above. Breathe in this way throughout the exercise.

- Starting with your hands, as before, extend the palm and fingers, then stop stretching and let your hands rest in your lap.
- Make sure that your elbows are not clenched tightly against your sides.
- Working up your arms to your shoulders, press your shoulders down away from your ears to prevent them being hunched up, then stop pressing – and notice the difference; you may need to do this movement two or three times to recognize the relaxation effect.
- Gently and slowly move your head from side to side, thereby stretching your neck muscles.
- With an open mouth, press your lower jaw downwards, then stop pressing and let your mouth almost, but not quite, close.
- Moisten your lips, teeth and the roof of your mouth – and smile!
- If you have not already done so, you might like to close your eyes and just enjoy the quiet and peacefulness.
- Keeping your eyes closed, raise your eyebrows towards the ceiling, then stop raising them and let your eyes rest.
- Imagine someone sweeping their hands gently up your forehead, drawing all the tension out of the top of your head.
- Working down your back, check your shoulders – and if necessary, press them downwards again, then stop pressing and recognize the relaxation.
- If necessary, adjust the position of your head and neck by gently moving your neck backwards and forwards.
- Press the small of your back into the support of the chair or bed, then stop pressing and adjust the position of your bottom.
- Make sure your thighs are not clenched tightly together; if you need to, place your thighs slightly apart.
- Roll your knees outwards and let them rest comfortably.
- Gently and slowly circle your ankles, first in one direction and then the other.
- Finally, pull your toes towards your nose (upwards), stop pulling and let your feet settle into a position that is comfortable for you.
- Check each of the muscle groups you have stretched to ensure they are all relaxed and rest for a few minutes, perhaps listening to some calming music.
- Throughout, remember to Sigh Out Slowly.

symptoms and discomforts of pregnancy

This chapter deals with the problems which occur in pregnancy due to the changes caused by weight increases and fluctuations in hormone levels. Most of these conditions are dismissed by doctors as 'minor disorders' of pregnancy, but for some women they can become major discomforts. If left unresolved, some of the conditions can worsen and develop into medical problems of pregnancy: I have therefore given guidance as to when to report the condition to your midwife or doctor so that the appropriate medical treatment can be provided at an early stage.

For each problem, I have provided several suggestions for steps you can take to help yourself – the majority of these involve the use of complementary therapies, while some are simply commonsense ideas.

These suggestions are followed by advice on how seeking expert assistance from a qualified complementary practitioner, where appropriate, may help to alleviate the symptoms.

nausea and vomiting

Sickness is often one of the earliest symptoms which may cause you to wonder if you are pregnant. It is an extremely common complaint, and may vary from mild nausea on waking to frequent vomiting throughout the day.

The hormones present in your body in the early weeks of pregnancy are notorious for making you feel sick as they affect your stomach, your appetite and the special centre in the brain which can trigger a vomiting response. Sickness is usually a sign that the hormone levels in your bloodstream are high enough to ensure that the pregnancy is well established: the sicker you feel, the higher the hormone levels. This is why women who are expecting more than one baby often experience worse sickness.

As the hormones settle down after about 12–14 weeks, most women find that the sickness reduces too, although this is not so for everyone as some mothers-to-be experience sickness throughout. A few women will experience a return to the nausea towards the end of pregnancy as the hormone levels change again in readiness for the birth. Hunger and tiredness can make the sickness worse. This is why many expectant mothers report early morning sickness when they wake up with an empty stomach; alternatively, tiredness at the end of the day can trigger early evening nausea.

When to seek further advice
If you are constantly being sick throughout the day and are unable to keep down any food you will eventually become dehydrated, and this will affect both your own health and that of your baby. If you vomit more than four times a day or the nausea continues past 20 weeks of pregnancy, you should consult your midwife or doctor.

Very occasionally, some women develop such serious vomiting that they require hospital admission. This is called hyperemesis gravidarum and treatment is by intravenous fluids to replace nourishment and fluid, and drugs to stop the vomiting. It is possible, however, to continue using complementary therapies alongside such treatment on condition that your doctor or midwife is aware of what you are using.

SELF-HELP

- **Nutritional therapy** Eat little and often to avoid over-filling your stomach at any one time.
  Eat a snack such as cereal or toast before going to bed; keep a couple of dry biscuits beside the bed along with a drink, in case you wake in the night or for the early morning. Maintain your blood sugar levels by snacking on high-protein and unprocessed carbohydrate foods such as oat or rice cakes, tahini, wholemeal bread, peanut butter, etc.
  Avoid those foods that are most likely to make you feel sick, eg fried, fatty or spicy foods.
  Discover (probably by trial and error) which foods and/or drinks help to relieve the sickness, eg crisp green apples, natural whole yogurt, fresh lemons or lime juice cordial.
  Sucking peppermints can be useful if you have nothing else to hand, but may not be as effective as some of the other remedies suggested.
  Reduce your intake of tea, coffee, alcohol and other stimulants, as these will inhibit the absorption of iron from your food and can lead to headaches, which compound the nausea.
  Supplements of vitamin B6 and zinc, as well as chromium, can be very effective, especially for women who were recently taking the contraceptive Pill as this impairs the body's ability to absorb these nutrients from the food you eat.
- **Herbal remedies** Try camomile or spearmint tea, or ginger tea made from grated ginger root steeped in boiling water, or ginger capsules available from healthfood stores.
- **Bach flower remedies** Use Rescue Remedy if you become anxious, especially if the anxiety makes the sickness worse.

- **Aromatherapy** Essential oils such as the citrus oils (orange, mandarin, lime, bergamot and grapefruit) are gentle and safe to use at this time. Add four drops of the oil of your choice, diluted in 5ml/1 teaspoon of carrier oil, to your bath, or put two drops on a cottonwool ball to sniff when you feel nauseous (this latter method is good for labour sickness, too). Peppermint or spearmint and ginger are also effective, but you will need to keep doses of these low enough so that you do not find the aroma overpowering, which in itself might make the nausea worse.
- **Acupressure** Try the 'sea sickness' wrist bands which are available at your local pharmacy or healthfood store. These work on the principle of acupuncture/acupressure (see page 28) and specifically on the acupuncture points at the P6 point on the inner wrists. Tiny acupressure magnets are also available, which are applied to the wrists with tape; although these coils are more expensive than the bands, they are usually more effective.

It is important to ensure that the bands or magnets are positioned correctly (see fig. 1, page 208) otherwise they will not work. To find the exact point on your inner wrist where you should position the button on the inside of the wrist band, or the magnet, use your own fingers to measure three finger-widths up on the opposite wrist: this is approximately where the buckle of a watch strap might rest. If you press firmly between the two tendons in the centre of the area you will feel a bruised sensation: the more nauseous you feel, the more bruised the point will be, and you will know you have found the correct spot!

There has been a lot of research into the use of acupuncture and acupressure to treat sickness, not only in pregnancy but also for people suffering vomiting after surgery or during cancer treatments with drugs or radiotherapy. Many of these trials have been carried out by doctors of conventional medicine and by nurses and midwives, and have proven repeatedly that these treatments can be equally as effective as medical drugs, but without the side effects. Some hospital departments now use acupuncture or acupressure as a cost-effective means of dealing with certain types of sickness.

Homeopathy

Take one 30C tablet of the most appropriate remedy every two hours, as required.

- If the nausea is constant and made worse by the smell of foods – ipecacuanha.
- If the sickness is worse in the morning – nux vomica; if it is worse in the evening, but better by night time – pulsatilla.
- If you constantly feel hungry but eating meat makes you feel worse – petroleum.
- If the sickness if accompanied by heartburn and diarrhoea – arsenicum.

OTHER THERAPIES WHICH MAY HELP

For these therapies, refer to a qualified practitioner.

Osteopathy or **chiropractic** can be used to realign your spine and release tensions which may be causing nausea, especially if you have a history of spinal or neck problems prior to pregnancy.

Acupuncture or **shiatsu** aims to rebalance the relevant energies, usually related to the Liver and Spleen, according to Traditional Chinese Medicine.

Homeopathy or **herbal medicine**, as it is important to ensure selection of the most appropriate remedy.

Reflexology can be used for general relaxation or for specific treatment of the foot zones which relate to the digestive tract. It is my experience that women who suffer severe sickness in pregnancy often have a history of neck injury such as whiplash or back problems, and that by using reflexology on the foot zones for the neck and spine, nausea and vomiting can be reduced.

Hypnosis may help to alleviate severe sickness. A trial in the 1980s explored the use of hypnosis for hyperemesis gravidarum and found that treatment was more effective when given to groups of women rather than to individuals.

Catherine's story

I saw Catherine in my clinic when she was nine weeks pregnant. Her nausea seemed to last all day and she was actually being sick at least twice a day, usually in the evening. She had previously tried ginger tea, to no avail. I suggested that she should try acupressure magnets over the P6 points on her wrists and the homeopathic remedy pulsatilla, one tablet three times daily for three days. As she was also very tired and stressed, I advised her to use the Bach flower remedy olive, two drops three times daily, and to relax in the bath each evening with essential oils of mandarin and lime, two drops of each in 5ml/1 teaspoon of carrier oil. Catherine reported that she had had bunions on the knuckles of her big toes operated on when she was 13, and on questioning her further it transpired that she had had neck problems ever since. As a reflexologist this was no surprise to me, for the areas of her bunions are the zones for the neck and upper back. I performed reflexology on her feet, concentrating on this area. Catherine telephoned me a few days later to cancel her next appointment, informing me that the sickness had all but stopped and she now only felt nauseous first thing in the morning.

appetite and taste, teeth and gums

You may have already noticed that your appetite and tastes have changed since you became pregnant, for either better or worse. One of the pregnancy hormones, oestrogen, is an appetite stimulant and you may therefore find that you develop a voracious appetite. On the other hand, sickness, anxiety or other symptoms may adversely affect your desire to eat, even if only temporarily. Changes also occur in your tastes, causing you to 'go off' certain foods or drinks such as tea or coffee, or to develop cravings for unusual foods.

This seems to be nature's way of telling you something. The foods that you no longer want are often those which are best avoided or reduced in pregnancy, perhaps because they are stimulants or can lead to potential problems for the baby – alcohol is an example. On the other hand, feeling a desperate need for one particular type of food may be a way of your body telling you that you are deficient in something. For example, a desire for strawberries could be due to a lack of vitamin C, a craving for grapefruit might indicate a need for vitamin B6, seafood and shellfish could signal a demand for zinc, and burnt toast might be a means of giving you extra carbon.

Cravings for unusual substances are very rare and often associated with other nutritional and/or emotional problems. I have looked after several women who have craved the smell of wellington boots or rubber tyres, and one mother-to-be who was so desperate for the smell of petrol that she carried a small bottle around with her!

You may find that the amount of saliva you produce is increased during pregnancy, although this does not normally become a major problem. However, very occasionally a woman may find that she produces so much excess saliva that she constantly feels the need to spit and has to carry tissues or a small pot with her at all times.

It is a fallacy that you lose a tooth for every child you have, because babies do not steal the calcium in your teeth until they are already very severely under-nourished: it is far more probable that they will use up the calcium in your bones first. The idea originated at a time when expectant mothers were generally less well nourished than they are now and had repeated pregnancies, and these factors combined to undermine general health and well-being. It is true, though, that teeth problems such as receding or bleeding gums can occur, and it is wise to obtain specialist dental advice during your pregnancy.

When to seek further advice

If you experience ongoing toothache or excessively bleeding gums, you should visit your dentist or inform your midwife or doctor – remember that in some countries dental care is free during pregnancy.

SELF-HELP

- **Nutritional therapy** A metallic taste in the mouth indicates a lack of zinc, and you should either eat plenty of foods which contain zinc – such as spinach, lamb chops, Brazil nuts, oysters or seaweed – or take a supplement.

  Drinking lemon or lime juice or sucking a piece of the fruit may remove some of the unpleasant tastes you develop in your mouth; if you have excess saliva, this may help to reduce the amount.

  Sucking peppermints may also help to remove unpleasant tastes. Peppermint toothpaste will freshen the mouth – be sure to use a toothbrush that is not too hard, and do not use peppermint if you are also using homeopathic remedies.

Try not to give in too much to cravings; instead, eat as well-balanced and varied a diet as you can, and consider also taking a good quality multivitamin and mineral supplement so that any deficiencies can be corrected.

- **Reflexology** The reflexology zones for the teeth are situated on the sides of the toes. If you experience an ache in a specific tooth, you can use reflexology as a 'first aid' technique by finding the relevant zone (left foot equals left side of the mouth) – the correct point will feel painful. Press firmly on this point until the pain under your thumb subsides, then repeat until your toe no longer feels painful – this will ease the pain in your tooth.

- **Aromatherapy** Essential oil of cloves, used neat and held in the mouth around the area of a painful tooth, acts as a pain reliever – but *do not swallow the oil*. Alternatively, you can use dried cloves and bite down on one or two held over the relevant tooth.

OTHER THERAPIES WHICH MAY HELP
For these therapies, refer to a qualified practitioner.
Hypnotherapy may be helpful in extreme cases of cravings, although usually these subside once the hormone levels settle down.

constipation

Many women experience constipation from an early stage of their pregnancy, as the hormones relax the digestive tract and slow down the movement of the intestines. The problem may be made worse if you have a tendency towards constipation when you are not pregnant; if you are unable to eat appropriate foods due to early pregnancy sickness; or if you are given iron tablets to combat anaemia, although these should not normally be given routinely. It is important to try to avoid constipation if you also have haemorrhoids (see page 91), as hard stools will make the piles more uncomfortable and may cause them to prolapse outwards.

When to seek further advice

If at any time you become very bloated and uncomfortable, or if you have not had your bowels open for more than a week, be sure to inform your midwife or doctor. If you experience headaches with the constipation, you may be being affected by the accumulation of toxins as a result of not emptying your gut, and this can eventually cause you to become unwell, so again, inform your midwife.

SELF-HELP

- **Nutritional therapy** Drink at least 3 litres of fluid daily, preferably water or fruit juice. If you drink a lot of tea, reduce this to less than three cups each day: tannin in tea (the component that stains the teapot brown) slows down the motion of the guts and increases the risk of constipation.
  Start meals with raw foods such as a salad or fruit. Eat foods which are rich in fibre (roughage) and also vitamin C – these include citrus fruits, blackcurrants, wholegrain cereals and bread, artichokes, celery, watercress and green vegetables.
  Use plenty of garlic in your food: peeled but not chopped whole cloves will ensure you obtain enough of the active ingredient without suffering the effects on your breath or an after-taste.
- **Aromatherapy** Add three to four drops of essential oil, diluted in 5ml/ 1 teaspoon of carrier oil, to your bath: citrus oils such as grapefruit, orange, mandarin or lime are good; marjoram can also help, but as this has a somewhat medicinal aroma you may wish to combine it with one of the citrus oils (to a maximum of four drops in total).
- **Herbal remedies** Try drinking mallow or dandelion root tea daily. Senna is a traditional remedy for constipation but is rather too purgative to use during pregnancy.
- **Reflexology** A simple home remedy is to ask someone to massage the arches of your feet in a clockwise direction: this is the area of the foot which relates to the intestines (see fig. 4, page 209) and working clockwise encourages movement of the bowel.
  You could also try rolling your foot arches over two bottles on the floor, which has a similar (though not so dramatic) effect.

- **Acupressure** Several times each day, press intermittently, about 20–30 times, on the CV6 acupuncture point, which is situated in the middle of your abdomen, about three finger-widths below your navel (see fig. 2, page 208).
- **Yoga** Positions can be learnt which may help to ease the discomfort caused by the constipation.
- **Massage** Working on your abdomen in a clockwise direction stimulates movement of the bowels; you could use plain carrier oil or add two drops of an essential oil such as bergamot or mandarin.

Homeopathy

Take one 30C tablet of the most appropriate remedy every two to four hours, as required.

- If the stools are soft despite the constipation and you feel that they are lodged in your rectum, and especially if you are better able to pass a motion when you are standing up rather than sitting on the toilet – causticum.
- If the stools are hard, smell sour and are covered with white mucus – graphites.
- If the stools are hard, cause you pain before passing them but leave you with an unfinished feeling – nux vomica or kali carb.

OTHER THERAPIES WHICH MAY HELP

For these therapies, refer to a qualified practitioner.

Osteopathy or **chiropractic** can be used to reduce tensions on the digestive tract and intestines and generally tone the body.

Acupuncture or **shiatsu** aims to encourage free-flowing energies along the relevant meridians.

Sarah's story

I saw Sarah in my complementary therapy antenatal clinic when she was 22 weeks pregnant. She was so constipated that she had not had her bowels open for three weeks and felt awful. I performed reflexology on her that day and again a few days later, and at her third visit she reported that she was now able to have her bowels open three times a week. A few weeks later, while Sarah was still attending my clinic weekly, I went on holiday for four weeks. When I returned, she was almost sitting on the doorstep waiting for me to do some more reflexology, for her constipation had returned with a vengeance! Again, after only two treatments she felt relieved, and I continued to see her weekly for the rest of her pregnancy to keep her constipation at bay.

headaches

Headaches are common in early pregnancy and are usually caused by relaxation of the blood vessels in the brain as a result of the pregnancy hormones, particularly progesterone. If you are feeling tired, nauseous or stressed, or have problems with your eyesight, headaches may be more frequent or more severe; if you have previously suffered from migraines, these can become more troublesome during the first three to four months of pregnancy.

When to seek further advice
Most headaches stop after a few (uncomfortable) months and severe headaches in late pregnancy are uncommon. However, headaches which occur in the last 12 weeks before the birth and which are focused around the forehead and over the eyes should be reported to your midwife or doctor. A relatively uncommon but potentially serious complication of pregnancy called pre-eclampsia can develop, which involves fluid retention, usually swollen ankles, high blood pressure and protein in your urine. In the early stages you feel well, but as the condition becomes more severe you may develop headaches and other symptoms (see Hypertension, page 132). In rare cases it can lead to fitting and jeopardize both your own health and that of your baby.

SELF-HELP

- **Aromatherapy** Use one drop each of neat essential oil of lavender and peppermint and rub them into your temples.
- **Acupressure** Locate the exact focus of your pain and press for two to three minutes on the spot: this is likely to be one of the relevant acupuncture points.
- **Bach flower remedies** If your headaches become worse when you are stressed or irritable, try impatiens for impatience, olive for tiredness, walnut to help you cope with the physical and emotional changes you are going through, or Rescue Remedy for generalized stress.
- **Herbal remedies** Those which may help include lavender or dandelion root tea.
- **Massage** Try using a 'hairwashing' movement over your scalp – make sure you are massaging the skin of your scalp and not just moving your hair over your head.
- **Nutritional therapy** Avoid caffeine and foods containing E additives where possible.
- **Yoga, Tai Chi** or **relaxation techniques** SOS – Sigh Out Slowly – breathing exercises (see page 66), dance and other forms of exercise may ease headaches caused by tension.
- **Reflexology** A simple technique is to view your two big toes as your head and neck, with the right big toe relating to the right side of your head and the left toe relating to the left side. The upper surface of your toes (with the nail on) is the front of your head and your face, and the back of the toes is the back of your head. Work out exactly where in your head the focus of the pain is and relate this to the position on your toes: for example, if the pain is over your forehead, the upper surface of both toes just below the nail will be the appropriate spot. When you have worked out the points on your toes, press on them with your thumb – this will feel painful, with either a sharp, needle-like pain or a dull bruised sensation, depending on how severe your headache is. Press on this spot until the pain beneath your thumb has gone, release and repeat until you toes no longer feel tender: this should have the effect of at least reducing the intensity of your headache, even if it does not ease it completely.

Homeopathy

Take one 30C tablet of the most appropriate remedy, as required.

- If the headaches are on the left side and over the eye – sepia, which is the most commonly effective remedy.
- If the headaches are worse in the evening – pulsatilla.
- If you become irrationally angry out of all proportion to the severity of the headaches – chamomilla.
- If the headaches are pounding, worse with jarring movement, and especially if you are pregnant during the summer months – belladonna.

OTHER THERAPIES WHICH MAY HELP

For these therapies, refer to a qualified practitioner.

Acupuncture may be used to encourage free-flowing energies along the relevant meridians.

Osteopathy or **chiropractic** works to reduce tensions in the neck and shoulders which can lead to headaches.

Hypnotherapy can be useful when the headaches are made worse by over-worrying and fear, possibly of labour.

insomnia and tiredness

Inability to get to sleep is common during pregnancy, as is waking frequently during the night. Often it is due to your mind remaining active and the feeling that you are not able to 'switch off' from the stresses of the day, especially when pregnancy and impending parenthood bring extra worries. It may be because you are physically uncomfortable – perhaps you need to get up to use the toilet several times, or your breasts hurt when you lie in certain positions, or you have backache. These discomforts can become worse as pregnancy progresses and may be exacerbated by the baby's movements which, while being exciting, can be very distracting at night. If you do manage to get to sleep you may experience vivid dreams, which are sometimes related to subconscious concerns about the baby or the birth.

Tiredness is almost universal, particularly in early pregnancy and again towards the end, initially as your body becomes accustomed to the circulating pregnancy hormone levels, then later due to the increased weight and problems with insomnia.

You may need to accept that rest and sleep must be obtained whenever they can, irrespective of the time of day or night: this is especially pertinent after the baby is born, when you will have to be up to feed him/her.

When to seek further advice

If you are unable to obtain adequate sleep and rest, your ability to cope with the physical and emotional challenge of pregnancy and your resistance to infection are lowered and you can become ill. You should therefore keep your midwife informed about your energy levels and your sleeping pattern. In severe cases you may need pharmaceutical drugs to enable you to rest and sleep.

SELF-HELP

- Although you should ensure that you drink plenty of fluids during the day, you could try having nothing further to drink after 7pm, so that your bladder is not over-full and you are (slightly) less likely to be woken by the need to use the toilet.
- **Relaxation techniques** Avoid all stimulants in the evening – these include coffee, tea, cola and chocolate, as well as heated discussions and noisy, exciting or violent television programmes (watching the news is not usually very relaxing!). Try listening to quiet music instead; if you use the same piece of relaxing music every time you will eventually develop a Pavlovian response to it – that is, it will act as a trigger to lull you to sleep.
  'Counting sheep' (visualization) is not as ridiculous as it sounds – you could try imagining yourself in a peaceful, beautiful countryside or beach setting or other scenario which conjures up feelings of tranquillity and joy for you. If you really cannot sleep, get up and do something – don't just lie awake worrying because you think you should be asleep!

Try combining the visions of tranquillity with SOS – Sigh Out Slowly – breathing (see page 66).

Make sure that you are well supported to obtain the most comfortable position. This is not so much of a problem in early pregnancy, although if you compress your breasts by lying on your front they can be tender; lying on your back may relieve the breast tenderness. However, this is not advisable in later pregnancy, when the weight of the heavy uterus presses on the big blood vessels returning blood to the heart and can lead to temporary dizziness and reduced oxygen supply to the baby. If your back aches and you lie on your side, it is important not to allow the knee of your top leg to fall forwards to rest on the bed, as this puts an extra twist on the small of your back. Put a cushion between your knees to keep your thighs parallel and another underneath your 'bump' for support. In later pregnancy, if you suffer from heartburn you may need to sleep propped up on at least two, if not three, pillows to prevent acid regurgitation.

- **Herbal remedies** Try sipping a cup of camomile or lavender tea before you go to bed. Herbal or hop pillows on which you rest your head can also be of use. An infusion of hops or skullcap just before retiring may aid the onset of sleep.

- **Aromatherapy** Essential oils such as lavender, camomile or ylang ylang in the bath may help you to relax – use four drops in 5ml/1 teaspoon of carrier oil; alternatively, one drop of neat lavender oil on your pillow will be relaxing. If you choose to use room vaporizers or burners, make sure you do not leave them burning (or plugged in, if electric) all night – your nostrils can only absorb a certain number of the molecules and continuing to use the oil all night is not only wasteful but can also be nauseating for some people (including your partner!).

- **Bach flower remedies** If you feel stressed and tense and your mind is over-active, try taking four drops of Rescue Remedy neat on your tongue before going to bed and again if you wake during the night. Two drops of olive taken in a small glass of water can also be helpful if you feel immensely tired but are still unable to sleep, and may also assist you to cope the day after a poor night's sleep.

- **Massage** Ask someone to massage your back, shoulders and neck just before you go to bed. Regular massages throughout pregnancy will relax you, encourage sleep and rest, and make you feel nurtured.

- **Yoga** or **Tai Chi** These therapies, plus relaxation or antenatal classes such as exercise-in-water, may ease your mental, emotional and physical stresses.

Homeopathy

Take one 30C tablet of the most appropriate remedy at night and then every hour if you are still unable to sleep, as required.

- If you experience nervousness, fear, restlessness, constant tossing and turning, and vivid dreams when you do sleep – aconite.
- If you have an over-active mind, experience over-excitement and euphoria, and if you sleep until about 3am and then are only able to doze – coffea; this is a particularly useful remedy if you are unable to sleep after the baby has been born because you are still 'on a high'.
- If you have an over-active mind, twitching limbs, sleep deeply but have nightmares and wake up jerkily or screaming – belladonna.
- If you experience a nervous irritation and itching of the upper body, sleep restlessly with constant murmuring, and dream of death and other disturbing possibilities – gelsemium.

OTHER THERAPIES WHICH MAY HELP

For these therapies, refer to a qualified practitioner.

Acupuncture or **shiatsu** aims to rebalance your Yin and Yang energies: this may be combined with suggestions for changes to your diet which can assist in the energy rebalancing.

Chiropractic, osteopathy or **cranial osteopathy** is relaxing and may relieve physical symptoms such as backache and heartburn.

Hypnotherapy in a more formal setting can be used to guide you through some of the imagery techniques and possibly help you to overcome specific fears, especially about labour or parenthood.

Reflexology performed regularly throughout pregnancy will aid relaxation and have a cumulative effect.

Alexander technique can re-educate your posture so that other aches and pains are reduced, thereby encouraging sleep.

stress, tension, anxiety and mood swings

Pregnancy is a time of immense emotional, physical and practical change; indeed, it is the single most important event in the lives of most people. Although the majority of women will be pleased that they are pregnant, even if initially it was a surprise, this is not necessarily the case for everyone. Even if the baby is much wanted and you are delighted to have conceived, you and your partner will have worries about numerous issues, which may not be the same for both of you.

Mood swings are common in pregnancy, as a result of fluctuating hormone levels and their effects on both your emotions and your physical condition. Stress may be exacerbated by everyday problems, especially if you have several other children to care for or are continuing to work. Emotional stresses can lead to physical tensions and add to the general discomforts of pregnancy; conversely, medical conditions arising during your pregnancy will aggravate your worries and concerns. It is not the purpose of this book to deal with the causes of all the emotional problems you may experience during your pregnancy, but complementary therapies can be extremely helpful in relieving the effects of some, though not all, of your anxieties and stresses at this time.

When to seek further advice

If either you or your family become aware that your behaviour is increasingly irrational, withdrawn or 'out of character' you should consult your midwife, health visitor or doctor. If you have a history of severe mood swings, depression or manic behaviour, you may be more prone to postnatal depression after the birth of this baby, but 'forewarned is forearmed' and appropriate steps to help you can be taken early.

SELF-HELP

- **Aromatherapy** Suitable essential oils for the bath, a room vaporizer or as a massage blend include ylang ylang, neroli, bergamot and lavender, which are all relaxing, or the citrus essences such as orange, mandarin, lime or grapefruit, which are uplifting. Use two drops in a vaporizer and four to six drops in 5ml/1 teaspoon of carrier oil for massage or to put in the bath.

- **Bach flower remedies** Suitable choices include olive to cope with general tiredness, hornbeam for a 'Monday morning feeling' of weariness, elm if you feel overwhelmed by responsibility or gorse for despair at your situation.

- **Nutritional therapy** A well-balanced diet is important, including plenty of fresh fruit and vegetables and not too many processed or 'instant' foods. A good multivitamin which contains zinc and vitamin B complex will assist with the absorption and proper utilization of nutrients from the foods you eat.

- **Tai Chi, yoga, relaxation** or **hydrotherapy classes** All these can help relax you physically, mentally and, if they are specific antenatal classes, enable you to meet other expectant mothers.

- **Herbal remedies** Try agnus castus tablets or jasmine tea. However, recent research appears to suggest that St John's wort, an excellent herbal antidepressant, should not be taken during pregnancy or breastfeeding; similarly passiflora, a herbal remedy for mood swings and insomnia, is contraindicated at this time. Spearmint or peppermint tea may lift the spirits, and burdock, blessed thistle or orange peel can help to maintain emotional balance.

- **Homeopathy** Remedies such as sepia if you are despondent or arnica if you are exhausted may be helpful.

OTHER THERAPIES WHICH MAY HELP

For these therapies, refer to a qualified practitioner.

Acupuncture or a complete **shiatsu** treatment will aim to rebalance your energies, relieve physical discomforts and stimulate and clear the meridians.

Osteopathy or **chiropractic** may be used to correct physical symptoms which may be adding to your general stress; **cranial osteopathy** can release tensions within your head which may be adding to your emotional state.

Alexander technique will help to correct your posture, which is affected by muscular tensions, and improve general health and well-being.

Massage, reflexology or **aromatherapy** can promote overall relaxation.

carpal tunnel syndrome

This condition can occur at any time during pregnancy but usually becomes worse in the last three to four months. It is due to swelling (oedema) such as you may develop in your ankles, but this occurs in your wrists and compresses the channel of nerves which runs up your arm. Pressure on the nerves causes a tingling, which sometimes becomes quite painful, and is often accompanied by loss of grip. It is worst when you first wake up, as your hands and arms may have been compressed as you slept. If you have experienced this problem in one pregnancy it is likely to recur in subsequent ones, and there is more risk of developing the syndrome in later life, unrelated to pregnancy.

When to seek further advice

Usually the condition will disappear once you have given birth to your baby, although despite doctors' reassurances that it should resolve dramatically within days it may persist for some weeks, possibly worsening temporarily in the first few days following delivery. If the problem continues after you have had your postnatal examination when the baby is about six weeks old, you should again consult your doctor, who may be able to refer you for a specialist medical opinion.

SELF-HELP
● Splinting your hands before going to bed may assist in preventing them from curling up while you sleep – your doctor, midwife or physiotherapist should be able to obtain some specially designed splints for you.

Alternatively, you can make your own by bandaging pieces of stiff card to your inner palms to prevent you from flexing your hands, although these are cumbersome and can cause difficulties if you have to get up to go to the toilet during the night.

- Try 'wrist wringing': clasping one wrist with your other hand and massaging it with a circling movement, similar to the 'Chinese burn' which you may remember from childhood; change over to the other hand after two to three minutes.
- **Aromatherapy** Essential oils which may encourage fluid dispersal include cypress or juniper berry, although you should not use the latter if you have any kidney problems; make a compress by soaking a cloth in water to which you have added four to five drops of the essential oil and wrap it around your wrists.
- **Herbal remedies** Camomile tea will encourage excretion of excess fluid.
- **Reflexology** Find the centre of the spot on the upper surface of the foot which relates to the wrist (see fig. 4, page 209) – it will be painful when you press it. Press on this spot until the pain beneath your finger disappears, and repeat until your wrists feel more comfortable. You will need to work on both feet if the problem affects both wrists.
- **Acupressure** Press firmly for seven to ten seconds, three times, on the P6 acupressure point on the inner wrists (see fig. 1, page 208).

Homeopathy

Take one 30C tablet of the most appropriate remedy three times daily for up to three days.

- If the tingling and numbness extend up your arm, your wrists and fingers are swollen, and the first and second fingertips of your left hand are the worst affected – apis.
- If the tingling and numbness extend to your shoulders and are worst in the fingertips of whichever side you are lying on – arsenicum.
- If the tingling is in your first, second and third fingers with swelling in your wrists – calcarea carbonica.
- If the wrist swelling happens in the evening, the pain is worst in your fingertips and in the evening and at night, and you have deformed and brittle nails – sepia.

OTHER THERAPIES WHICH MAY HELP

For these therapies, refer to a qualified practitioner.

Acupuncture or **shiatsu** can be applied to specific points which act as a first aid treatment to relieve intense pain.

Osteopathy or **chiropractic** works to realign any minor spinal deviations, especially in the neck vertebrae, and to release tensions in the wrists.

backache and sciatica, pubic and coccyx pain

Many women experience backache at various times during pregnancy, especially if they have had problems beforehand. This is partly due to the pregnancy hormones which relax the joints, ligaments and muscles in the pelvis in preparation for labour, but is compounded by the increasing weight as the baby gets bigger. This often has the effect of making you stick your abdomen out, thereby increasing the curve in the small of your back. Lower backache is most common, although pain in the upper back, neck and shoulders may occur either due to stress or, after delivery, as a result of the position you assume in order to feed the baby.

Sciatica occurs when the sciatic nerve, which runs down from the pelvic area to the leg, becomes irritated and/or compressed and you experience a sharp, shooting pain intermittently down your leg. Occasionally you may find your leg 'gives' under you as you walk and causes you to stumble. This will also occur if you suffer from ligament pain, which arises as the hormones stretch the ligaments that hold the pelvis and pelvic organs in place.

Pain in the pubic area can be due to a condition called symphysis pubis diastasis, a separation of the cartilage which holds together the two pelvic bones that meet in the middle of the pubic area. It has only been recognized as a fairly serious condition in recent years, despite many women having complained of severe pain in the pubic region. It, too, is due to the effects of hormones but some women seem more prone to it than others. Walking becomes extremely difficult and the pain can be made worse by prolonged sitting or standing, or lying in one position for too long.

Localized pain may occur in the region of the coccyx (tailbone), perhaps if there is a history of a previous fall or a difficult delivery in an earlier pregnancy, which may have caused a very fine fracture in the tiny bones that make up the coccyx.

When to seek further advice

Doctors can be notoriously dismissive of back pain during pregnancy, but you should ask for a referral to a physiotherapist if the sharp, shooting pains persist or you find walking and moving increasingly difficult. Probably the most effective treatment is either osteopathy or chiropractic, and it may be possible for you to be referred by your doctor or to obtain such treatment via private medical insurance. The effect of hormones on your muscles and skeleton means that it can take up to a year following the birth for your spine, bones, muscles and joints to return to the normal non-pregnant state, so care should be taken with lifting and carrying, especially as your baby grows bigger and more mobile.

SELF-HELP

- Think 'tall': imagine balancing a book on your head, which should encourage you to straighten the curve in the small of your back.
- Make sure your shoes are comfortable and that the heels are broad and not too high – you may have to surrender vanity to comfort!
- Prioritize your household chores – let someone else do the heavy jobs if at all possible; balance shopping bags evenly in both hands to avoid overweighting one side; after the birth, as your baby grows, avoid carrying him/her on one hip.
- Sleep well supported by cushions or pillows: if you lie on your side, ensure that the thigh of your top leg remains parallel to that of your underneath leg – place a pillow between your thighs and one in front of your knees to avoid your leg falling forwards to rest on the bed. After delivery, use plenty of pillows to support yourself and the baby while

you are breastfeeding – bring the baby up to your breasts rather than bending down to him/her.

- **Massage** Ask someone to rub your back *gently*, which may provide temporary relief. It is important to avoid pressing too deeply into the hollows of the sacrum in the small of the back, as there are acupressure points here which can stimulate the onset of labour. If you also have sciatica, it is wise to avoid massage until the cause of the pain is known.

- **Aromatherapy** Essential oils added to your bath are relaxing and offer some pain relief: lavender and marjoram contain chemicals which are known to be pain-relieving, while ylang ylang, petitgrain or neroli are generally relaxing. Marjoram is good for muscular pain, and rosemary may help if you have sciatica, although this should not be used if you have high blood pressure. Use a maximum of four drops of essential oils in any preferred combination, diluted in 5ml/1 teaspoon of carrier oil.

- **Bach flower remedies** Rescue Remedy cream rubbed into the area may help. If tiredness increases the discomfort, use two drops of olive in water, three times daily or as required.

- **Herbal remedies** A compress of mustard flowers steeped in warm water and applied via a cloth to the affected area can relieve some of the pain.

- **Yoga, Tai Chi** or **relaxation exercises** These will increase your mobility and suppleness – try also pelvic rocking, lying on your back with your knees drawn up and rocking from side to side.

- **Hydrotherapy** This is beneficial in that it encourages greater flexibility and movement; if you enjoy swimming this can also help, but you must be careful to avoid arching your neck – if using breast stroke, make sure your face goes in the water so that your spine remains straight.

Homeopathy
Take one 30C tablet of the most appropriate remedy, as required.
- If the backache is due to trauma such as a fall, feels bruised and sore to touch, and extends to the pubic bone and the joints at the back of the pelvis – arnica.
- If the pain is in the small of the back and of sudden onset, causing a dragging sensation, and is worse if there are any jarring movements – belladonna.
- If there is numbness in the back but sciatica runs from the hip down the outer

sides of the thighs, especially on the right side, and makes you feel completely worn out – phytolacca.

- If you have a bruised, aching, dragging sensation in the small of the back and it is associated with constipation – nux vomica.
- If the pain is in the small of the back or lower, and between the shoulder blades, feels like a burning sensation and as if the back is broken, is worse when getting up from sitting and causes you to feel weak – phosphorus.

OTHER THERAPIES WHICH MAY HELP

For these therapies, refer to a qualified practitioner.

Osteopathy or **chiropractic** would be my personal recommendation for serious back, neck and pelvic problems. Research has shown that chiropractic is especially good at treating symphysis pubis diastasis. Pain in the coccyx can be treated by osteopathy but treatment may need to be performed via the rectum to be most effective, so you will need to consider whether or not this is acceptable to you.

Reflexology can be generally relaxing and may reduce some of the discomfort; it is particularly effective in reducing neck pain. Pain which originates in the joints at the back of the pelvis (the sacroiliac joints) can be eased using reflexology, but relief will be temporary as reflexology cannot treat the cause.

Acupuncture or **shiatsu** can be used to encourage the production of the body's own natural pain-relieving chemicals and rebalance energies which may either have caused the problem or arisen as a result of it.

Alexander technique is a more long-term commitment to improved posture.

haemorrhoids

Haemorrhoids (piles) are varicose veins in the rectum and anus which occur during pregnancy because the hormones relax all the veins in the body. They are very common and usually manifest themselves towards the end of pregnancy, when the increased weight from the baby is pressing down and the pelvic floor muscles in the area between the vaginal opening and the anus are relaxing. They are likely to be worse if you are expecting more than one baby or have put on a lot of weight, or if you have had them before, either in a previous pregnancy or at other times. Some women find that the haemorrhoids are just slightly uncomfortable after defecating, perhaps itching or with occasional bleeding, while for others they are distinctly painful all the time; having the bowels open, or the action of pushing the baby out for delivery, can cause the veins to prolapse so that they protrude outwards and look like a large bunch of grapes.

When to seek further advice

In almost all cases, haemorrhoids disappear within six to eight weeks following delivery as the hormone levels return to normal. However, if they continue to cause you pain, particularly if they have prolapsed outwards, it is best to consult your doctor; occasionally, very severe haemorrhoids require surgery to remove them, although this would not be performed during pregnancy.

SELF-HELP

- **Nutritional therapy** Avoid constipation by eating high-fibre foods and plenty of fruit and vegetables, and drinking copious amounts of water and fruit juice, but avoid too much tea and milk, both of which may exacerbate the constipation (see also Constipation, page 76).
- **Relaxation techniques** When you are sitting on the toilet, try to breathe deeply, then exhale and relax your pelvic floor muscles but take care to avoid straining. You could also try a standing position, perhaps with one knee bent and your foot on a stool (or on the bath, if it is in a suitable position), as this encourages relaxation of the pelvic floor and opens up the area more than sitting with your buttocks clenched.
- **Herbal remedies** If the haemorrhoids protrude and are painful, you could apply witch hazel lotion to them or add it to a bidet for use after having your bowels open.
- **Aromatherapy** Cypress or frankincense essential oil added to the bidet or used as a compress on a sanitary towel acts as an astringent to tighten the protruding veins. Use four drops of essential oil in 5ml/ 1 teaspoon of carrier oil.

- **Bach flower remedies** Add four drops of crab apple to the bidet; if the haemorrhoids are not bleeding, you could rub Rescue Remedy cream into them to bring relief.
- **Shiatsu** Apply 'first aid' to the GV20 point on the top of your head (see fig. 3, page 208) – ask someone to press firmly on this point for seven to ten seconds, three times.

Homeopathy

Take one 30C tablet of the most appropriate remedy every two to four hours for up to three days, as required.

- In the absence of any more specific remedy being indicated – pulsatilla; this is a fairly universal remedy for haemorrhoids and works especially well for women who also have varicose veins and/or heartburn.
- If the haemorrhoids are bluish/purple, large, congested, bleeding and extremely painful, but improve from bathing in warm water – arsenicum.
- If the haemorrhoids are large, congested, grape-like, bleeding, protrude when either having the bowels open or passing urine and a stitching sensation is felt in the rectum when coughing – kali carb.
- If the haemorrhoids are large, grape-like, congested, protruding and painful; where there is associated constipation with hard stools and backache, but the pain is better from bathing in cold water – nux vomica.
- If the haemorrhoids are large, hard and grape-like, protrude during defecation, itch and bleed with continual oozing and there is a sensation of a hard ball in the rectum – sepia; this is a good remedy for haemorrhoids which occur or continue to be troublesome after delivery.

OTHER THERAPIES WHICH MAY HELP

For these therapies, refer to a qualified practitioner.

Acupuncture will focus primarily on the UB57 point on the back of the calf (see fig. 4, page 209) – often one treatment is enough to ease the discomfort.

Shiatsu aims to rebalance the Spleen and Bladder energies and promote a general feeling of relaxation.

Reflexology can be applied to the specific foot zone for the rectum, plus general work to stimulate the bowels and avoid constipation.

heartburn and indigestion

Heartburn, indigestion and oesophageal reflux of acid may develop in late pregnancy, as a result of relaxation by hormones of the valve at the top of the stomach which allows some of the acid stomach contents to flow back up the oesophagus (gullet). The problem may be exacerbated by pressure from the baby as s/he pushes up under the ribcage and diaphragm before dropping down to become engaged in the top of the pelvis, and it may also be worse if you are expecting more than one baby. Certain foods will make the heartburn more acute.

When to seek further advice

If, after trying a range of complementary therapies, you still obtain no relief, or if the condition is so severe that it begins to affect your everyday life, it is wise to consult your midwife or doctor, who may be able to prescribe drugs to suppress the effects of the acid reflux. Usually no further treatment is recommended during pregnancy, but if the problem persists for several weeks after delivery you may have a more serious condition such as hiatus hernia, which may require surgery.

SELF-HELP

- **Nutritional therapy** Avoid tea, coffee, alcohol, sugar and E additives, especially E276; trial and error will highlight which foods are best avoided, but fried or spicy foods are frequent culprits. Remember that smoking will aggravate your symptoms.
  Try eating small, frequent meals to avoid over-filling your stomach with one large meal.
  Raw garlic eaten daily or garlic capsules can help combat indigestion.
- **Herbal remedies** Ginger, dandelion root or camomile tea, or slippery elm tablets, may be beneficial. Caraway, dill or fennel seeds added to cooked food will act directly on the digestive tract to regulate acidity.

- **Aromatherapy** It is worth trying four drops of lemon, orange or neroli with one drop of oil of black pepper in 5ml/1 teaspoon of carrier oil, either in a massage to the chest and upper back or in the bath.
- **Shiatsu** Apply 'first aid' to the P6, St36 and CV22 points (see figs 1, 2 and 4, pages 208–9): press intermittently 20–30 times every couple of hours.
- **Yoga** or **Tai Chi** classes can teach postures and positions which may help to alleviate some of the discomfort.

Homeopathy

Take one 30C tablet of the most appropriate remedy every two hours, as required.

- If the heartburn is worse after eating and causes you to 'burp', leaving a metallic taste; your stomach feels bloated, cramping, heavy and sore – nux vomica.
- If the heartburn is worse after supper, drinking milk, eating rich, fatty food, fruit, meat or bread; 'burping' gives you a taste of the food you have just eaten or a slimy, salty taste in your mouth; your stomach feels empty and gurgles and rumbles in the evening – pulsatilla.
- If 'burping' gives you a rancid taste in your mouth; you feel nauseous and bloated; you have pressing stomach pains and the heartburn is worst in the morning or after eating rich or fatty foods – carbo veg.

OTHER THERAPIES WHICH MAY HELP

For these therapies, refer to a qualified practitioner.

Acupuncture or **shiatsu** can be applied specifically to the Stomach meridian to rebalance energies.

Osteopathy or **chiropractic** may be used to release tensions in the chest.

Reflexology can help if applied to the foot zones related to the oesophagus and top of the stomach.

Alexander technique can help by encouraging a more upright posture, which reduces tension around the area of the stomach and oesophagus.

ankle oedema (fluid retention) and leg cramps

About 50 per cent of pregnant women develop fluid retention in late pregnancy, usually in the ankles and feet, but also in the fingers, wrists (see Carpal tunnel syndrome, page 86), face and other areas. It occurs due to congestion caused by pressure which prevents free flowing of the circulation.

The filtering system of the kidneys is not as efficient in pregnancy as normal and also interferes with the body's ability to excrete excess fluid. This is seen most markedly after delivery, when swollen ankles can temporarily become much worse. This is because all the extra tissues which were developed to grow and nourish the baby during pregnancy are no longer required and are dissolved and excreted via the kidneys as urine. However, the kidneys are unable to deal efficiently with all the extra fluid and some collects in the areas surrounding the blood vessels until the kidneys are ready to excrete it all. Sometimes the swelling can be so marked that it stretches the skin of the lower legs, which becomes shiny, taut and very uncomfortable. In Traditional Chinese Medicine terms, oedema is seen as a depletion of energy in the Spleen and Kidney meridians, energies which naturally decline with age, so pregnant women over the age of 35 may experience worse swelling and fluid retention than younger mothers.

Leg cramps often occur during the night when you are curled up in bed and are related to salt levels and changes in the circulation. Traditional Chinese Medicine also sees the cause as related to a deficiency of Blood and Kidney energies.

When to seek further advice
Swollen ankles are not usually considered by doctors to be a problem in pregnancy unless they are accompanied by excessive swelling elsewhere in the body, raised blood pressure and protein in the urine, all of which amounts to the condition of pre-eclampsia which can lead to fitting (see Hypertension, page 132). If you experience headaches,

visual disturbances or pain in the upper right-hand side of your abdomen, you should consult your doctor or midwife without delay for further investigations.

SELF-HELP

- Towards the end of pregnancy, rest with your legs up as much as possible: this will not only encourage you to rest generally but, in Traditional Chinese Medicine terms, will improve the flow of energy along the Kidney meridian, which easily becomes depleted through inadequate rest.
- To save yourself money, avoid wearing too many different pairs of shoes in late pregnancy, especially leather ones, as these will stretch and be too large once you have had the baby.
- If swelling occurs in your hands and fingers, be sure to remove rings before they become too tight – if you leave them, they may have to be cut off in order to prevent loss of circulation.
- If you suffer cramps, refrain from adding extra salt to your meals as this may increase your risk of fluid retention. When cramp strikes, stretch the leg or foot as much as possible to prevent muscular contraction.
- Rest the arches of your feet on two bottles and roll them backwards and forwards on the floor, to increase circulation to your legs and feet and stretch the calf muscles.
- **Herbal remedies** Wrap a compress of cabbage (dark green is best) or geranium (*Pelargonium*) leaves around your legs – wipe but do not wash them and cool them in the fridge, then wrap the leaves firmly around your legs. Leave them until they become wet, then replace with others until you feel some relief from the swelling.
- **Massage** Ask someone to massage your legs upwards from foot to knee (or thigh, if the swelling is severe) with both hands, using vegetable oil, talcum powder or soap and water as a lubricant. This will disperse the fluid upwards, and although only temporary it will give some relief.
- **Aromatherapy** Rest your feet in a foot bath to which you have added essential oils of cypress, juniper berry, geranium, rosemary or patchouli (a maximum of four drops in total).

- **Bach flower remedies** Add two drops of olive and four drops of Rescue Remedy to a foot bath if your legs feel tired.
- **Nutritional therapy** Increase the use of onions, parsley and garlic in your food and reduce the amount of unrefined carbohydrate, all of which will aid excretion of excess fluid.
- **Yoga** or **Tai Chi** Attending classes may help.
- **Hydrotherapy** Swimming, or pregnancy classes which offer exercise in water, can be pain-relieving, reduce swelling and relieve cramp.
- **Shiatsu** Apply 'first aid' for cramp by pressing the UB57 point on the back of the calf (see fig. 4, page 209).

Homeopathy for cramp
Take one 30C tablet of the most appropriate remedy, as required.
- If the cramp is worse in the evening and when you stretch yourself out in bed – chamomilla.
- If the cramp occurs during labour – nux vomica.
- If the cramp happens in late pregnancy while you are walking, and you are snappy, worn out and have no appetite – sepia.

OTHER THERAPIES WHICH MAY HELP
For these therapies, refer to a qualified practitioner.
Homeopathy for the oedema, so that the full symptom picture can be obtained and an appropriate range of remedies prescribed.
Acupuncture or **shiatsu** may be used to stimulate the Kidney and Spleen energies for oedema and the Bladder meridian for cramp.
Reflexology combined with foot **massage** will encourage improved circulation and more efficient working of the kidneys, as well as relieving the acute, painful swelling of the ankles and lower legs which can occur in late pregnancy or the early postnatal period.
Alexander technique can re-educate your posture and improve circulation.
Osteopathy or **chiropractic** can be used to relieve any restrictions in the ankle, knee and hip joints and to stretch relevant muscle groups.

sinus congestion, coughs and colds

Respiratory problems can, of course, occur during pregnancy as easily as at any other time and are usually seen as coincidental to the pregnancy. However, in Traditional Chinese Medicine theory these problems, particularly chronic coughs, are thought to be due to weakened Kidney energy, which leads to weakness in the lung area. The traditional encouragement to drink plenty of milk is actually inappropriate in today's well-nourished society, although many expectant mothers still believe they should do so, but dairy produce is well documented as increasing mucus production, so anyone with a tendency to sinus congestion is likely to be more seriously affected.

Although, on the whole, coughs, colds and sinus congestion are not problems which require medical attention, they often initiate other symptoms such as headaches, and excessive coughing can lead to a feeling of straining around the abdominal area. If a cold or cough develops, it is acceptable to use small amounts of most of the popular medicines for these conditions, although it is wise to read the label before taking anything. If you prefer not to take pharmaceutical drugs, there are a few strategies using natural remedies which may help.

When to seek further advice

If your symptoms do not subside, and particularly if your temperature remains raised, you may have influenza or another respiratory infection. Continued high temperatures may lead to premature labour in susceptible people. Minor 'flu-like illnesses can also be a sign of a relatively rare infection such as toxoplasmosis, which is acquired through contact (usually unknown) with cat faeces and which, if contracted in early pregnancy, can cause abnormalities in the baby. It is therefore important not to ignore ongoing 'flu symptoms.

SELF-HELP

- **Aromatherapy** Essential oils such as tea tree, eucalyptus, frankincense or naiouli are safe to use in small doses in pregnancy and can ease congestion and fight infection. Put two drops of any of the oils on a tissue or add to a bowl of hot (not boiling) water to use as a steam inhalation with a towel over your head. Alternatively, if you have a burner you could add two drops to vaporize into your room. If you also have a sore throat, the two drops of essential oil can be added to 5ml/1 teaspoon of carrier oil and rubbed into the skin of your throat, as well as over your chest and back. The choice of oils will depend on your personal preference, but the total number of drops should not exceed two, used about every four hours. You could also relax in a bath to which you have added about six drops in total: this could be a blend of several of the oils already mentioned. Research has indicated that eucalyptus appears to be safe to use throughout pregnancy; tea tree similarly is considered to be an extremely versatile and safe oil. Lavender oil helps ease congestion as it is an expectorant, although its use in very early pregnancy is still under debate; there are many different types of lavender oil and some are potentially more liable to trigger vaginal bleeding if used to excess.
- **Herbal remedies** Peppermint or dandelion root tea may ease some of the 'blocked-up' feelings.
- **Massage** Working on the head and face, focusing on the scalp and under the cheek bones, can be relaxing and effective in clearing the sinuses.
- **Reflexology** Use this to work on the points on the feet related to the face (see fig 4, page 209). Otherwise, simple foot massage, working on the upper surfaces just below the toes and on the balls of the feet, will suffice.
- **Nutritional therapy** Avoid too many dairy products to discourage production of extra mucus. Short-term high doses of vitamin C are thought to enhance the immune system, but their use is controversial and it is best to obtain your vitamin C through eating plenty of citrus fruit or drinking the juice. However, zinc lozenges are safe and effective in boosting the immune system, and zinc can also be taken in the food you eat – lamb chops, dark green vegetables and Brazil nuts are all good sources.

- **Relaxation techniques** Deep breathing exercises can assist in clearing the respiratory tract and encourage use of the base of the lungs which may feel compressed, especially in late pregnancy when the baby is pushing up under your ribcage.
- **Shiatsu** Suitable techniques include applying pressure to the relevant acupuncture points on the head and around the eyes: these will normally feel tender at this time, so are relatively easy to find by gentle probing along the upper edges of the ridges of the eyes.

OTHER THERAPIES WHICH MAY HELP
For these therapies, refer to a qualified practitioner.

Shiatsu or **acupuncture**, working along the length of the Kidney meridian, can stimulate increased energy flow and reduce breathlessness.

Osteopathy or **chiropractic** can realign the skeleton to reduce chest tensions.

varicose veins

Like haemorrhoids, varicose veins in the legs are common in pregnancy because the hormones relax the walls of the blood vessels, causing the veins to 'kink' and the valves inside them to become inefficient. Varicose veins can also occur in the vulval area, around the opening to the vagina. The veins often throb, especially as the increasing weight of the baby presses downwards, and gravity intensifies this feeling. If you are expecting more than one baby, are overweight, have had several full-term pregnancies or are over the age of 35 you may be more at risk of varicose veins, especially if you have had them before or in a previous pregnancy.

When to seek further advice
Most women find that varicose veins disappear within six to eight weeks following delivery, although this is not always the case. In pregnancy, it is important to ask your doctor or midwife to examine the area of your legs where the varicosities are situated to ensure that

they are not becoming ulcerated or threatening to develop into thrombosis. It is particularly relevant that the midwife who delivers your baby is aware of vulval varicosities, because there may be a need in labour to perform an episiotomy (a cut to enlarge the vaginal opening) which can increase the risk of haemorrhage in the area. If at any time your legs become hot, painful and red in one isolated area you *must* inform your doctor. If the varicose veins have not subsided by the time the baby is six weeks old, you may need to be referred to a specialist surgeon.

SELF-HELP

- Rest with your feet up as much as possible to reverse the effects of gravity.
- Avoid carrying things which are really heavy, especially if you have vulval varicosities. Try wearing double sanitary pads in your underwear to provide support underneath and reduce the feeling that everything is 'falling out'.
- **Massage** Avoid working on areas where there are varicose veins, as it is possible tthat this could cause trauma which may dislodge clots and lead to thrombosis.
- **Bach flower remedies** Two drops of olive, three times daily or as required, may ease some of the weariness which can increase the discomfort from varicose veins in both legs and vulva – either take this by mouth or add it to a shallow bath.
- **Herbal remedies** A witch hazel compress – a cloth soaked in cold water with a few drops of witch hazel lotion added – on your legs acts as an astringent and encourages constriction of the blood vessels; for vulval varicosities, put the witch hazel in a shallow bath and sit in it for ten minutes. Yarrow tea may also help – sip a cup two to three times a day.
- **Aromatherapy** Sitting in a bath with added essential oils of cypress, juniper berry and/or lemon has a similar effect and is relaxing, but do not use juniper berry if you have a history of kidney disease; use four drops in total in any combination, diluted in 5ml/1 teaspoon of carrier oil. You can freshen your feet and legs by soaking them in a bowl of cool water with two drops of peppermint oil added to it, or combine the oil with body lotion to rub into your legs.

Homeopathy

Take one 30C tablet of the most appropriate remedy three times daily for up to three days, as required.

- In the absence of any other symptom picture suggesting a different homeopathic remedy – pulsatilla, notably in women who are also suffering heartburn; alternatively, hamamelis could be used.
- Varicosities which cause heaviness, are worse in the morning and make you snappy and indifferent – sepia.
- Vulval varicosities which throb, ache and feel bruised, are worse on the left side and if you become overheated – bellis perennis.
- If your varicose veins are painful, possibly ulcerated and affected by extremes of temperature – lycopodium.
- If the varicosities feel sore and burning, are worse when you are cold, and you feel anxious, sluggish and have difficulty concentrating – calcarea carbonica.

stretch marks, itching skin and eczema

Stretch marks seem to be the bane of every pregnant woman's life. You may reach almost the end of your pregnancy without developing any, then be disappointed to find them in the last two weeks before the birth. They mainly occur on the abdomen, inner thighs and buttocks, but may also appear on the breasts. It depends on the elasticity of your skin, notably the layer underneath the top layer, as to whether or not you will develop them, but despite numerous suggestions from both commercial pharmaceutical companies and advocates of complementary medicine, it is difficult to prevent them. If stretch marks are going to happen they will, and women who are carrying a very big baby or more than one are more likely to develop them because their skin needs to stretch more to accommodate the pregnancy. Although stretch marks are often quite vividly red during pregnancy they usually fade to a silvery colour after delivery, but unfortunately they are permanent.

Itching skin occurs in late pregnancy in about 17 per cent of expectant mothers and is usually related to salt levels in the blood, but may also be triggered by infections, certain drugs, allergies or eczema. Often the itching is around the abdomen, or it may be localized in specific areas – for example, if it is due to thrush the vaginal region will be irritated and sore, or it may be seen in an area exposed to something to which you have developed an allergy.

Eczema is a stress-induced condition which may already be present when you conceive and may get better or worse during pregnancy; some women find that it occurs for the first time during pregnancy. Anxiety will certainly exacerbate the condition, so any complementary therapy which reduces the impact of stress can be helpful. (For advice on coping with more acute eczema, see page 127.)

When to seek further advice

If the itching is due to a skin rash, you should consult your doctor as you may have contracted an illness such as chickenpox which will require attention. If you develop itching accompanied by yellowing of the skin (jaundice), you *must* inform your doctor. An extremely rare but serious liver complication of pregnancy is often preceded by intense itching of the skin and it will be necessary to take blood from you to test that your liver is functioning properly.

SELF-HELP

- **Herbal remedies** Camomile lotion acts as a cooling agent to prevent you from scratching your skin too much.
- **Homeopathy** Chamomilla may decrease the irritation; take one 30C tablet every two hours.
- **Aromatherapy** Cool baths containing four to six drops of essential oil of lavender or camomile in 5ml/1 teaspoon of carrier oil will ease pregnancy itching. A good regime for eczema is to use the oils in the bath in rotation over a three-week period – one week of lavender, one week of camomile and one week without. If there is a rash you could try four drops of tea tree oil, but be aware that a few people find tea tree oil irritating in itself.

- **Massage** Giving your abdomen a massage with a very rich carrier oil such as avocado with wheatgerm will nourish the skin and may reduce the incidence of stretch marks.
- **Bach flower remedies** Rescue Remedy cream applied to the worst areas of itching or eczema can reduce the intensity of the irritation. Two drops each of impatiens, crab apple and star of Bethlehem diluted in 250ml of water and applied to the skin as a compress may also help.
- **Relaxation techniques, Tai Chi** and **yoga** All these may aid relaxation if stress, anxiety and tension are exacerbating your skin problem.

OTHER THERAPIES WHICH MAY HELP
For these therapies, refer to a qualified practitioner.

Acupuncture or **shiatsu** can be effective in treating itching skin and eczema.

Homeopathy may eventually treat the cause, particularly if you have eczema which was present before conception. However, eczema is such a complicated condition that it is difficult to elicit the cause and very careful monitoring by the homeopath will be needed.

Hypnotherapy has been found to be effective in reducing the itching associated with eczema and in modifying allergic responses.

vaginal discharges and urinary symptoms

Vaginal discharge usually increases during pregnancy due to increased blood supply, which leads to an increase in mucus production from the cervix and to a change in the pH balance of the lining of the vagina. This is called leucorrhoea. It should, however, remain the normal whitish colour, be non-irritant and have no unpleasant odour. Pregnant women are prone to thrush, which is caused by a yeast-like fungal infection that flourishes in the more acid environment of the vagina during pregnancy.

Most women complain of an increased need to pass urine, especially in the first three months of pregnancy when the growing uterus presses on the bladder, before it becomes too large to occupy the pelvic cavity and moves upwards into the abdominal cavity. Towards the end of pregnancy, when the baby's head engages and drops below the level of the top of the pelvic bones, there is further pressure on the bladder and, according to all the books and magazines you might read (including professional textbooks for midwives and doctors!), the need to pass urine frequently returns. In truth, the majority of expectant mothers will experience this frequency throughout pregnancy, due to downwards pressure and the relaxation of the pelvic floor muscles and sphincter from the bladder. The bladder is also less able to retain as much urine as you would normally expect, so that when you do go to the toilet there is merely a 'dribble'. As with vaginal discharge, however, there should be no change in colour or odour and no irritation.

Very occasionally a condition arises at around 16–20 weeks of pregnancy in which, because the uterus is tilted backwards, it has difficulty in rising out of the pelvic cavity into the abdominal cavity. This has a knock-on effect in that the bladder becomes trapped by the growing uterus, which results in an inability to pass urine until the bladder is over-full, which then further prevents the uterus from rising upwards. Medical treatment for this condition, which is called retroverted incarcerated gravid uterus, involves the insertion in the vagina of a special plastic ring to make the uterus tilt forwards, so that it can then rise up into the abdominal cavity and release the trapped bladder.

When to seek further advice
If your vaginal discharge causes itching either internally or outside the vagina, if it becomes creamy, grey, greenish or blood-stained, or if it develops an unusual odour you may have an infection which will need to be treated before you go into labour. Most vaginal infections are eminently treatable, but if left untreated can be passed to the baby as s/he travels down the birth canal which may affect his/her eyes, mouth or digestive system.

If you experience difficulty in passing urine, if it causes a stinging or burning sensation either as you pass it or immediately afterwards, or if it changes colour or odour you should also seek help, as this could be a urinary tract infection. Cystitis is simply inflammation of the bladder but does not necessarily mean there is an infection, although it may go on to develop into one. This can be treated with antibiotics which are safe to take during pregnancy, but if left untreated can trigger premature labour or track upwards to the kidneys, leading to more serious kidney problems.

SELF-HELP
- Take care with personal hygiene, keeping the whole area clean and uncontaminated, especially after having your bowels open – if you have a bidet, it is a good idea to get into the habit of using it regularly. Avoid perfumed soaps, detergents and vaginal deodorants.
- **Nutritional therapy** You should reduce your intake of refined carbohydrates and foods which contain sugars, including the 'hidden' sugars that are found in savoury products such as baked beans or tomato ketchup. Keep your alcohol consumption down to the minimum, because its sugar content will increase the risk of infections, either vaginal or urinary.
  Eat a diet rich in vitamins and minerals, including plenty of fruit and vegetables, and consider taking a supplement with zinc, iron and vitamin C. Good quality natural yogurts with acidophilus help to maintain an appropriate pH of the vagina, reducing the risk of thrush. Eat plenty of raw garlic.
  You should aim to drink at least 3 litres of water each day.
- **Aromatherapy** Adding essential oils to your bath (use four drops in 5ml/1 teaspoon of carrier oil) will help prevent both vaginal and urinary infections, as all essential oils are anti-infective in some way. If you are unable to bathe, keep a jug specially for the purpose and use it to pour water with essential oil added over your vulval area – you can sit on the toilet to do this. Particularly good oils for this purpose include tea tree, sandalwood, camomile or bergamot; use four drops in total in about 1 litre of cooled water.

- **Herbal remedies** A good preventative remedy is to drink a small glass of cranberry juice daily, which has been found to have an effect on the urinary tract. You must ensure that it is pure cranberry and does not contain any sugar, which will aggravate cystitis. Camomile tea is also a good urinary antiseptic.

OTHER THERAPIES WHICH MAY HELP

For these therapies, refer to a qualified practitioner.

Reflexology can be effective in encouraging the flow of urine when the bladder is trapped by a backwards-tilting uterus, so that there is then more space for the uterus to move up into the abdominal cavity.

Homeopathy for frequent passing of urine

Take one 30C tablet of the most appropriate remedy every two hours for three days, as required.

- If the urge to pass urine is painful and constant, and there is a burning pain during and after passing urine which is often involuntary, especially when you cough or laugh – pulsatilla.
- If you find yourself involuntarily passing urine while you sleep but there is a loss of sensation when you do pass urine – causticum.
- If the urge to pass urine is constant with a dragging pain in your pelvis, and it is difficult actually to start passing urine which is then dark, cloudy and contains sediment – sepia.
- If passing urine is involuntary and profuse, you experience a sensation of motion in your bladder and the urine is dark, turbid and contains blood for which no medical cause has been found – belladonna.
- If your bladder feels paralysed, passing urine causes a burning sensation and a feeling of weakness in your abdomen, and the urine is scanty – arsenicum.

problems with sex

Your desire for sex during pregnancy can be affected negatively or positively. Tiredness, nausea, aches and discomforts, vaginal discharges and anxiety about the baby can all conspire to reduce your desire for full sexual intercourse almost to nothing, although you may desperately feel the need for emotional intimacy with your partner. Conversely, and strangely, the removal of any risk of becoming pregnant can, for some women, increase their libido, particularly as the increased blood supply to the vagina and cervix heighten sensation and can make it easier to reach orgasm. Indeed, for some women who have never achieved climax, pregnancy can be the first time they experience orgasm.

Your partner may also find his sexual desire changes. Some men adore the sight of their partners when pregnant, others find it a big 'turn-off'. Many men have unnecessary fears regarding the effects of intercourse on the baby and the pregnancy, without perhaps realizing that the baby is contained within his/her own bag of fluid which cannot be reached by the man's penis or fingers being in his partner's vagina. Finding the time and opportunity to have sex is important – remember that you started out as a couple and, for most, having a baby is the culmination of your love for each other.

Following the birth you may reject full intercourse for several weeks due to the presence of vaginal blood loss, cuts, bruising or stitches. However, it is wise to have attempted some form of vaginal penetration before the sixth week, when you may be due to have a medical examination to ensure that your body is returning to normal. Problems arising at this time may identify any internal stitches which have not yet dissolved. (See also Care of your perineum, page 181.)

When to seek further advice

If you experience pain on intercourse, it may be wise to ask your doctor or midwife to examine you to ensure there is nothing physical which could be causing the problem. If your dislike or lack of desire for sexual intimacy becomes so overwhelming that it begins to affect your emotional relationship with your partner, enquire about specialist counselling. Relationship counselling or referral to a sex therapist may be necessary if the situation continues.

TIPS FOR IMPROVING INTIMACY

- Talk to each other about any fears or concerns you may have; ask your midwife or doctor for advice if necessary. If the person you speak to is unable to help directly, they should be able to refer you to someone who is better qualified to assist you.
- Consider ways of achieving intimacy without full penetrative sex – kissing, cuddling and mutual masturbation.
- Try different positions to accommodate your increasing size and changing shape – lying on your side or rear entry removes pressure on your abdomen; sitting astride your partner on a chair reduces friction on the walls of the vagina.
- **Massage** Use aromatherapy essential oils such as sandalwood, patchouli or ylang ylang, which are aphrodisiac, for a massage that is relaxing, soothing, intimate and a wonderful means of 'setting the scene' – try four drops in 5ml/1 teaspoon of carrier oil – or share a bath together.
- **Bach flower remedies** The choice will depend on the precise nature of your emotions, but possible remedies might include olive for tiredness, mimulus or larch for anxiety, agrimony if you constantly put on a brave face or holly for suspicion and jealousy.
- **Homeopathy** If you have lost all enjoyment of sex, have a strong aversion to it and a very dry vagina which itches and burns, especially if accompanied by a negative outlook – graphites. If you have no desire and don't even like the smell of your partner, sex causes vaginal pain and orgasm is painful – sepia or natrum mur. Take one 30C tablet of the most appropriate remedy three times daily for three days, as required.
- **Relaxation techniques** These could help if you become very tense just prior to penetration, especially if you are anxious about potential pain (see 'Private and personal', page 190).
- **Tai Chi, yoga** or **exercise classes** These will increase the level of endorphins and encaphalins produced from the brain, which will boost your sense of well-being.

Ellie's story

Ellie was a police officer with a demanding job, which she was now finding stressful and tiring as she was 20 weeks pregnant. She came to my clinic as she had told her own midwife that she was suffering from insomnia. She certainly looked tired, but while we were talking I sensed there was more to her situation than she had revealed. In the course of the conversation I asked a discreet question about her sex life which prompted a flood of tears, and she told me that her libido, which was normally good, was at an all-time low, yet her partner was very highly sexed and she was worried that she would lose him if they did not continue their active sex life during the pregnancy. We talked for a little longer and arranged a plan of relaxing aromatherapy and reflexology treatments to take her through the rest of her pregnancy.

Ellie agreed to try the Bach flower remedies olive for tiredness and hornbeam for weariness, elm to reduce the feeling of being overwhelmed at work and centaury to help her feel able to say 'no' occasionally. I also gave her a blend of carrier oil with essential oils of ylang ylang and sandalwood to use for massage or in the bath, and taught her some deep breathing exercises. Each week when Ellie came for her relaxation session we continued to talk, and this in itself seemed to help her to put the issue into perspective. The relaxation techniques appeared to be helping; after four weeks she no longer felt the need to discuss her sex life and we used the time to talk about other things, but continued with the reflexology and aromatherapy.

OTHER THERAPIES WHICH MAY HELP

For these therapies, refer to a qualified practitioner.

Reflexology or **shiatsu** treatments on a regular basis can increase your overall sense of well-being and relaxation.

Acupuncture can rebalance energies to stimulate the production of endorphins and encephalins, the body's own natural uplifting chemicals.

Hypnotherapy may be useful if the problem is long term and associated with fears and inhibitions. Although the problem may have been present before, it could be that pregnancy offers an opportunity to discuss it with a health professional, who can refer you or recommend you to a hypnotherapist.

4

illness in pregnancy

Pregnancy and childbirth are normal life events and usually proceed without major problems, apart from the physical discomforts that occur as a result of changes in your body (see Chapter 3). Very few expectant mothers require admission to hospital during pregnancy and about 75 per cent of births are normal, without complications. Occasionally, however, pregnant women become ill or develop problems during this time which require medical care. These problems might be:

- Illnesses which could occur at any time, but because you are also pregnant may need additional care. These include influenza, appendicitis, and kidney or urinary problems.

- Conditions which existed before conception and which may or may not worsen as a result of the physical stresses of pregnancy. These include anaemia, diabetes, asthma and eczema.
- Complications which develop as a direct result of being pregnant. These include vaginal infections, high blood pressure, vaginal bleeding or multiple pregnancy.

Some of these conditions fall into more than one category: for example, you may have high blood pressure before you become pregnant but the effects of hormones, increased weight and other factors exacerbate the problem and lead to the pregnancy-related complication of pre-eclampsia.

Complementary medicine offers a wide range of strategies for dealing with various medical conditions, but should be seen as just that – *complementary* to conventional treatment, an adjunct to orthodox management of the complications of pregnancy and childbirth. Such therapies can provide a means of relieving the different symptoms associated with medical complications, whether these arise as a result of the pregnancy or are incidental to it.

You have every right to administer natural remedies to yourself, but should keep your midwife and obstetrician informed so that they can work with you to provide the most appropriate care, and to avoid interactions between any necessary drugs and the remedies you choose to use. You may wish to consult a complementary practitioner as an alternative to medical treatment, especially if you have been seeing an individual therapist regularly. However, if you develop complications, whether they are pregnancy-related or a worsening of an existing problem, I would advise you to consult only those practitioners whose therapies are considered to be systems of medicine in their own right. These are homeopathy, acupuncture, osteopathy, chiropractic and herbal medicine, all of which are able to work at a deeper level than some of the more supportive therapies, although this latter group can provide some additional methods of easing your discomforts. If you are in any doubt, you should consult all the health professionals who are involved in your care – conventional and complementary. By asking questions, requesting advice and seeking clarification of information given to you, you should be able to make a judgement, in partnership with the team, about the most appropriate treatment for your particular situation.

This chapter focuses on some of the ways in which you may be able to use certain aspects of complementary medicine alongside any conventional medical treatment required for complications during pregnancy, in order to ease your discomforts and improve your sense of well-being.

influenza

The common cold was dealt with in Chapter 3 as a reasonably normal condition which can be self-medicated, irrespective of whether or not you are pregnant (see Sinus congestion, coughs and colds, page 99). However, influenza is a more serious condition which occasionally requires hospital admission, even in normally fit, healthy people. If you are also pregnant, your body is already working hard and, depending on your general health, you may be more susceptible to a cold which does not readily respond to the usual treatments. Influenza is caused by a virulent virus but antibiotics will not treat the problem, merely combat superimposed infections that you may contract as a result of being generally more susceptible.

When to seek further advice
It is important that influenza is not left to become more serious while you are pregnant because it may lead to miscarriage, or, if you develop an excessively raised temperature in later pregnancy, to pre-term labour, as well as undermining your general health and making you more likely to develop other problems. If the following self-help ideas do not bring down your temperature or make you feel better, you should consult your family doctor for more conventional treatment.

SELF-HELP

- **Aromatherapy** All essential oils are anti-infective, and most are capable of reducing the adverse effects of bacteria. Tea tree is renowned as a particularly good antiseptic, antiviral and antibacterial oil. You could use three to four drops in a vaporizer to help you breathe; it may also help to reduce your temperature and combat the virus responsible for the influenza, as well as other infections caused by bacteria. The newer oils of manuka and kanuka from New Zealand are thought to be even more effective, but may be difficult to obtain. If you are able to get up to have a bath, put four to five drops of essential oil in the water; alternatively, you could ask someone to prepare a steam inhalation for you. Frankincense is also good as it helps you to cough up any phlegm and is relaxing. A single drop of black pepper oil added to the blend may help to reduce your temperature.
- **Nutritional therapy** Ensure that your diet contains plenty of garlic, or take good quality supplements. If you have been prescribed antibiotics to deal with any superimposed infection, take a course of yeast-free acidophilus with bifidus capsules and vitamin C (1g daily for a week) to prevent additional problems such as vaginal thrush. Eat plenty of fresh fruit and vegetables, and drink vast quantities of water.
- **Herbal remedies** Echinacea has been well researched as a means of preventing infection, particularly respiratory tract infections, and can also be taken in the event of actual illness.

operations during pregnancy

Occasionally problems occur that are unrelated to your pregnancy but require treatment by surgery, such as removal of your appendix. In other situations, an operation may be necessary because of a condition occurring during pregnancy: for example, removal of retained products following inevitable miscarriage (see Vaginal bleeding, page 137). Complementary therapies can be of use before the operation to de-stress and prepare you for the procedure, and afterwards to help you overcome the effects of the surgery, the anaesthetic and any pain.

SELF-HELP

- **Bach flower remedies** Rescue Remedy is extremely useful if you are very anxious and experience feelings of panic. Four drops can be taken neat on your tongue as required, even if you are not allowed to eat or drink anything else. Mimulus may reduce fear – take two drops neat or in a small amount of water, up to three times daily. If the need for surgery causes you extra worry about your family, especially if you have other children to take care of, take two drops of red chestnut, three times daily. Walnut is effective in helping you cope with changes that may need to take place while you recover. Once you are allowed up, crab apple can be added to your bathwater, to help ease any feelings of uncleanliness.

- **Homeopathy** Remedies which may be useful to combat the effect of drugs used during or after the surgery are detailed opposite.
  Arnica is a universal remedy which combats shock, trauma and bruising, and although research trials have been inconclusive, many people have reported that it lessens the impact of surgery and encourages a faster recovery. Similarly, hypericum has been used for wound healing. If these are used in the 30C strength (or 100C if you can get it), the suggested regime is shown opposite.

- **Aromatherapy** It is not possible to use essential oils around the time of the operation as they may interfere with drugs you need; being volatile, they may also cause environmental problems in the operating theatre when mixed with anaesthetic gases. However, essential oils can be very pleasant in helping you through the recovery phase following the surgery, both for relief of pain and to aid wound healing. Lavender oil is known to contain chemicals which are pain-relieving and, although research seems to indicate that its wound-healing capabilities are not as good as was once thought, it acts as an antiseptic and thereby can aid wound healing by preventing infection. Once your wound is uncovered and you are able to have a bath, you could add to the water two drops of lavender essential oil together with two drops of tea tree, which will also help to fight any infection. Camomile oil will enhance relaxation and make it easier for you to rest, and the citrus oils are generally uplifting and will cheer you up.

- **Herbal remedies** Marigold tincture can be applied to a wound and comfrey is well known as a good wound healer.

- **Relaxation techniques** Deep breathing exercises are fundamentally important following a general anaesthetic, to ensure that you utilize the full extent of your lungs and to prevent chest infection. SOS – Sigh Out Slowly – breathing may help calm you at any time before, during or after the operation (see page 66).
- **Acupressure** If you suffer from sickness after you 'come round' from the anaesthetic, try using wrist bands or acupressure magnets (see Nausea and vomiting, page 71).
- **Nutritional therapy** It is essential to maintain a nourishing diet to aid the healing process after surgery. Zinc is particularly useful for this and can be found in parsley, potatoes, garlic, carrots, beans, steak and lamb chops, nuts, egg yolk, rye and oats. Plenty of fluids in the form of water and fruit juice will flush out your system and prevent urinary infections, especially if you needed to have a catheter inserted in your bladder during the operation. Vitamin C and the B complex are also essential – if necessary, take a comprehensive multivitamin and mineral supplement to counteract any deficiency. In addition, it is important to take steps to prevent anaemia, which is more likely to occur if you have lost a lot of blood (see Anaemia, page 121).

Homeopathy

To reduce the effects of drugs used during surgery: take one 100C or 30C tablet of the most appropriate remedy three times daily for three days.

- If you have had a general anaesthetic which makes you feel 'spaced out' and dreamlike – opium, especially if the drowsiness is made worse from being over-warm. Opium is also useful if you have been given strong painkillers such as morphine or pethidine.
- If you feel euphoric but 'spaced out' and vomit bile while recovering from the general anaesthetic – phosphorus.
- If pethidine or morphine is given for pain relief following the operation and you are irritable, perspiring, intolerant and self-pitying – chamomilla.

After surgery, arnica and hypericum may aid recovery.

- Take one 100C or 30C tablet of each before the operation if possible – this will not compromise the fact that you will not be able to eat or drink anything.

- For the first 24 hours following surgery, take one tablet of each every hour (while awake).
- For the second 24 hours, take one tablet of each every 2 hours.
- For the third 24 hours, take one tablet of each every 3 hours.
- Stop after the third day.

OTHER THERAPIES WHICH MAY HELP

For these therapies, refer to a qualified practitioner.

Hypnotherapy has been used on a few occasions for relatively minor operations instead of a general anaesthetic, but you would need to find an extremely competent practitioner.

Acupuncture can be effective in relieving sickness and will help to accelerate your recovery period by rebalancing your energies. Acupuncture has also been used as an alternative to anaesthetic, mainly in China, but could potentially offer an opportunity to avoid the effects of the powerful drugs that are used to render you unconscious.

Osteopathy or **chiropractic** can be beneficial following surgery, particularly if you have ongoing aches and pains associated with the operation. These might be the local pain of healing in the relevant area, for example around a wound, or problems such as backache as a result of the position you were in during the operation. This is likely to be significant if you have undergone an operation performed vaginally for which you have been put in the lithotomy stirrups with your legs up, as this position can lead to misalignments of your spine in the following days and weeks.

Reflexology or **massage** can provide relaxation and pain relief following surgery and may help to prevent other after-effects of the operation such as constipation (see page 75).

kidney and urinary problems

Cystitis and minor urinary tract infections are covered in Chapter 3 (see page 105). However, occasionally more serious renal problems can occur during pregnancy or may exist before conception.

Pyelonephritis is a bacterial infection which affects the kidneys and upper part of the ureter, the tube that leads from each kidney to the bladder. Normal pregnancy changes in the kidneys and ureters mean that some women are susceptible to this condition, especially if there is a history of previous recurrent cystitis or other urinary problems. One of the most common bacteria to cause the infection is found in the intestines, while other bacteria flourish in the rectal area. If you develop pyelonephritis you will become quite seriously ill, usually in mid-pregnancy. You will have a high temperature, severe loin pain and headache. Your urine may be reduced in amount and will smell offensive. Hospital admission, bed rest and high doses of antibiotics are the normal treatment; if left untreated, you may develop fits and your baby may need to be delivered prematurely.

If you have an ongoing renal (kidney) condition from before you became pregnant, it is most likely that you will already be receiving strict medical care, and once you are pregnant, medical supervision will be increased.

The advice that follows looks at the ways in which complementary therapies can be used as a preventative measure against pyelonephritis, or used safely for general relaxation by women with severe renal problems. *It is inappropriate to consider their use as the only means of treatment.*

SELF-HELP

- **Aromatherapy** You can use essential oils in your bath or bidet to ensure total cleanliness after having your bowels open, as inefficient cleansing can encourage the passage of bowel and intestinal bacteria to the opening of the urethra (from which urine is ejected) or, indeed, into the vagina. Tea tree, lavender or sandalwood can be chosen; use a maximum of four drops in total of any of the suggested oils, diluted in 5ml/1 teaspoon of carrier oil. If infection occurs, try a compress of sandalwood and/or benzoin pressed against the small of your back or over your pubic area. Use four drops in 250ml of boiled, cooled water, then soak a cloth, wring it out and apply it to your chosen area. If you have a high temperature, add an additional drop of black pepper oil to the water.

- **Nutritional therapy** Maintain your body's ability to fight off infection by eating plenty of foods which contain zinc, vitamin C, selenium and garlic, or take appropriate supplements. Avoid acidic foods, which can aggravate any inflammation of the urinary tract caused by the infection.
- **Relaxation techniques** Keeping relaxed and calm helps to lower your blood pressure, which can rise in conjunction with renal disease; it will also aid your ability to resist infection. Try gentle exercise such as Tai Chi, as well as therapies such as aromatherapy, reflexology and acupressure.
- **Acupuncture** Chinese herbs or dietary adaptations, in line with Traditional Chinese Medicine to rebalance your body's Yin and Yang state, will render you less likely to succumb to major infections.
- **Herbal remedies** Echinacea may help to prevent infections generally. Dandelion tea acts as a good anti-infective agent. Drinking copious amounts of camomile tea will not only flush out the urinary tract but also reduce inflammation in the area, as 60 per cent of the chemicals in camomile are anti-inflammatory.
- **Hydrotherapy** Sitting in a bath or splashing water around the vulval area from a bidet can ease the irritation which you may feel at the opening to the urethra and bladder. If you are confined to bed you may welcome a 'wash down' with water, perhaps with the addition of the relevant essential oils, while sitting on a bedpan so that the water can be poured over your vulva. If you are able to obtain bunches of fresh camomile, add these while putting in the hot water, then cool with the required amount of cold water.

OTHER THERAPIES WHICH MAY HELP

For these therapies, refer to a qualified practitioner.

Osteopathy or **chiropractic** can be used if you have a history of kidney problems either before pregnancy or during a previous pregnancy. An osteopathic or chiropractic 'overhaul' can ensure that your joints, muscles and bones in the area of the kidneys are in alignment so that abnormal tensions are not placed on the urinary tract, predisposing you to infection during this pregnancy.

Reflexology given carefully by an experienced therapist can safely be used to aid relaxation and encourage the passage of urine; this can be used as a preventative measure and, with caution, if you actually develop the infection.

anaemia

Anaemia is a deficiency in either the quantity or quality of the red blood cells which carry oxygen around your body in the form of haemoglobin; this in turn leads to a reduction in the capacity of the red blood cells to transport oxygen to both you and your baby.

Iron is required for the production of enough good quality red blood cells, which is why pregnant women were traditionally given extra iron tablets to maintain their stores. However, in pregnancy various natural changes occur in your blood and it is normal for your haemoglobin levels to fall slightly, particularly in the middle months because there is a greater increase in the fluid than in the number of red blood cells, causing a dilution of the blood. It is therefore now generally considered unnecessary to give you iron tablets routinely unless investigations of your blood indicate the need to do so. However, your iron levels may already be low before you conceive, perhaps if you have had exceptionally heavy periods or several pregnancies close together, when there is insufficient time for your iron stores to recover in between.

You may suffer from an ongoing type of anaemia, which may not be iron deficiency but could be due to lack of the folic acid that is needed for formation of nuclei in all cells in the body. Another type of anaemia develops if there are inadequate amounts of the vitamin B complex to maintain the shape of the red blood cells. Some women, notably but not exclusively from specific racial groups, have a genetic disorder such as sickle cell disease or thalassaemia which also results in anaemia. It is not the intention of this book to deal with these last two types, and most women who have these conditions will already be under extremely vigilant medical care. Many of the self-help ideas which follow could, however, be used by anyone suffering from anaemia, whether this has arisen before or since conception.

In the early stages of anaemia you may look pale with dark rings under your eyes and you will feel immensely tired. It is essential that anaemia is diagnosed as soon as possible and treated before the birth, as the amount of blood lost during delivery may have a far greater effect on your health than the same amount of blood lost by a mother who is not anaemic.

When to seek further advice

If you feel continually exhausted and incredibly weary, or if you become very breathless, your iron stores may be very low and you should seek medical advice. Untreated anaemia leads to a reduced ability to cope with infection, a greater risk of thrombosis and lower oxygen supplies to your baby, resulting in poor growth and development.

SELF-HELP

- **Nutritional therapy** Diet plays a large part in increasing and maintaining your stores of iron and folic acid. Vitamin C is important to encourage absorption by the digestive tract of the iron you have consumed in food; it is found in all citrus fruits, many vegetables, blackcurrants, kiwi fruit, potatoes, rosehips, melon, parsley and fruit juices. Vitamin B complex is found in red meats, wholegrain cereals, brewer's yeast and vegetable proteins. Folic acid is found in green leafy vegetables, wholegrain cereals, eggs, liver and kidneys. For a comprehensive list of foods which contain iron, see opposite.
  Avoid foods which may interfere with your body's ability to absorb the relevant nutrients from your food. These include bran, tea and coffee.
- **Herbal remedies** A herbal tea made from yellow dock root, freshly picked nettles, parsley or peppermint may help.
- **Breathing exercises** Severe anaemia will make you more than usually breathless, so it is important to practise deep breathing exercises several times a day in order to inflate your lungs fully and enable them to work to their optimum capacity.
- **Aromatherapy** Although essential oils cannot prevent anaemia, it may be possible to reduce the risks of infection which can arise by using the notably anti-infective oils regularly. Tea tree, lavender, frankincense, naiouli, manuka and eucalyptus are all good for this, while one small research trial has suggested that lemon oil can increase white blood cell production to help prevent infection. Try a maximum of four drops in

total of any of the suggested essential oils, diluted in 5ml/1 teaspoon of carrier oil.

- **Bach flower remedies** The most appropriate remedy will probably be olive for the tiredness you feel – two drops in water, three times daily. However, you may also find other remedies useful, such as oak if you 'soldier on' to fulfil your responsibilities and fail to slow down for the sake of your own health. If you are a total perfectionist and find it difficult to accept help from others you could try beech, or vervain if your perfectionism has caused you to push yourself too far. If the thought of work, chores and the day ahead causes you unutterable weariness, hornbeam is the appropriate remedy.

Foods containing iron

- Whitebait, sardines in tomato sauce, sprats, kippers, pilchards, cockles, salmon
- Red meats, liver, egg yolk
- Red kidney beans, chick peas, soya beans, lentils
- Prunes, dried apricots, dried figs, dried peaches
- Spinach, seaweeds, watercress, dandelion leaves, chicory
- Potatoes, spring onions, parsley, chives
- Almonds, sprouted grains and seeds
- Wholemeal bread, wheat cereals, muesli
- Oat cakes, malt bread, molasses
- Chapatis, curry powder
- Ground ginger, ginger biscuits, ginger bread

OTHER THERAPIES WHICH MAY HELP

For these therapies, refer to a qualified practitioner.

Acupuncture or **shiatsu** may revolve around treating the symptoms of anaemia, such as working on the Kidney meridian for the breathlessness and the Spleen meridian for the tiredness. Acupuncture can cause changes in the way in which chemicals are used in the body and it has been used successfully to treat low haemoglobin levels. One study divided women who were found to be anaemic after the birth into three groups to receive either no treatment, iron tablets or acupuncture. When blood tests were taken after five days, results from

the women in the group who had received acupuncture were equal to those in the iron medication group, demonstrating the effectiveness of the acupuncture. **Homeopathy** may also be helpful. The remedy of choice depends on the nature of the symptoms and is best determined by a qualified practitioner.
Reflexology may be beneficial in easing the breathlessness, relaxing you sufficiently to induce sleep, or possibly in stimulating the immune system to prevent infection.

diabetes mellitus

Diabetes is a condition in which, due to an enzyme deficiency, inadequate or even no insulin is produced from the pancreas, which then affects the body's ability to metabolize sugars from the foods you eat. Insulin is needed to facilitate the conversion of these sugars into energy. Without insulin, this conversion cannot occur, the levels of unused glucose rise in your blood and some is excreted in your urine. Your body also attempts to use fats and proteins for energy, which in turn leads to the release of urea and ketones (waste products) into your urine. If you produce too many ketones, your body becomes very acidic and you can go into shock – a diabetic coma.

Some women develop diabetes in childhood and are therefore likely already to be under medical care, requiring insulin injections several times daily. If you are an insulin-dependent diabetic you may have had some difficulty conceiving in the first place but, once pregnant, may find that the two conditions have an adverse effect on each other: control of the diabetes becomes more difficult because of the pregnancy, and complications of pregnancy are more likely because of the diabetes. In this case, it is almost certain that you will already be under the care of specialist obstetricians and physicians, because the diabetes becomes very unstable during the pregnancy and you are likely to require more insulin.

Some women have diabetes before becoming pregnant but do not require insulin injections, possibly only tablets. However, the interactive effects of the pregnancy and the diabetes are similar to those in women with insulin dependency and you may need insulin injections for the duration of the pregnancy and through the early postnatal period.

During pregnancy it is also possible to develop a temporary gestational diabetes. The filtering action of the kidneys is not as efficient as when you are not pregnant, and the first indication of pregnancy diabetes is that a routine urine test shows glucose (sugar), although this does not necessarily mean that you have the condition. Women who are overweight, consume vast quantities of sugar-laden foods or are over 35 are more prone to this form of diabetes, as are women expecting more than one baby or whose baby weighs more than 4.5kg. Insulin injections or tablets are usually unnecessary, but you would be wise to be booked to have your baby in a specialist medical centre where any potential complications can be diagnosed and treated early.

Some of the complications of diabetes during pregnancy include an increased risk of vaginal and urinary infections (see pages 105 and 129) due to the sugar levels in the urine; more severe nausea and vomiting in the first three months (see page 69); high blood pressure and pre-eclampsia (see Hypertension, page 132); excessive fluid around the baby, causing greater movement within the uterus and the possibility of the baby being in the wrong position at the time of the birth; and a large baby which may become obstructed as s/he attempts to negotiate the pelvic canal during delivery. All obstetric care is geared towards preventing or minimizing the effects of these problems, but at the same time complementary therapies can also offer a way of assisting in this process.

When to seek further advice

If you are already aware that you are diabetic when you become pregnant, it is most unwise not to consult your family doctor, physician or obstetrician, although you may wish to continue to receive complementary treatment alongside conventional care. If at any time you suffer a diabetic coma, either from having too much sugar or not enough, you will need to receive emergency treatment at the time and then follow-up.

SELF-HELP

- **Aromatherapy** You can use essential oils such as lavender or ylang ylang to keep your blood pressure within normal limits and to relax you when you are anxious about your own health or that of your baby. Citrus oils, ginger or peppermint can decrease the severity of early pregnancy sickness. Sandalwood or bergamot in your bath may relieve cystitis and tea tree can treat vaginal thrush. You could try a maximum of four drops in total of any of the suggested essential oils, diluted in 5ml/1 teaspoon of carrier oil.

- **Nutritional therapy** Keep sugary foods to a minimum, including those savoury foods that contain 'hidden' sugars, to avoid both putting on too much weight and absorbing too many sugars with which your body may be unable to cope. Eat good quality carbohydrate foods for energy – bananas are a good emergency standby. Maintain fluid levels by drinking plenty of water. Some research has shown that eating foods rich in pyridoxine – vitamin B6 – can reduce the rate of complications from pregnancy diabetes. B6 is found in meat, fish, egg yolk, wholegrain cereals, avocados, bananas, grapefruit, nuts, seeds and leafy green vegetables. Reduce salt intake and, of course, alcohol consumption.

- **Massage** Asking your partner to massage your back, shoulders or feet can be very relaxing and will help to prevent excessive use of insulin through stress.

- **Tai Chi, yoga** or **relaxation exercises** These can assist in keeping you as fit as possible without undue strain on your insulin needs.

OTHER THERAPIES WHICH MAY HELP

For these therapies, refer to a qualified practitioner.

Osteopathy or **chiropractic**, being manipulative therapies, are not usually used to treat diabetes, although some practitioners may attempt direct treatment to the pancreas. However, if you are an insulin-dependent diabetic and choose to consult an osteopath or chiropractor for any reason, you should check your insulin levels after treatment. This is because the treatment has a similar effect to undertaking exercise and can alter your insulin requirements.

Reflexology can be relaxing, but it is important to consult a practitioner who understands the processes involved in pregnancy diabetes. If you are diabetic and wish to receive reflexology, the therapist should take care not to over-stimulate the area of the foot which relates to the pancreas, as this may change your insulin requirements. This applies at any time, not merely when you are pregnant.

asthma, eczema and hayfever

Although these three conditions are all very different, they are essentially problems which arise as a result of allergic responses to various substances.

Asthma is a condition which leads to recurrent attacks of wheezing, coughing, shortness of breath and a sense of suffocation, and is made worse by stress. Often it has been present since childhood. Many women experience fewer asthmatic attacks while they are pregnant, although this is not always the case. If you are asthmatic, you may be more likely during pregnancy to suffer from severe nausea and vomiting (see page 69), pre-eclampsia (see Hypertension, page 132) or bleeding (see page 137), and if you have frequent attacks of breathlessness your baby may be slow to grow. It is normal for medical treatments to be continued during pregnancy if you are severely asthmatic, including the use of steroids. One of the main ways in which complementary therapies can be of use is by helping you to relax, to prevent some of the triggers taking effect and to avoid over-breathing during an attack.

Eczema is a serious allergic skin condition which is often passed down through families. It may become worse or may improve during pregnancy. Some women who have not suffered before can develop eczematous rashes during pregnancy which are extremely irritating. If you have eczema your baby has a high risk of developing the condition, especially if given cow's milk. Stress very definitely exacerbates the condition. (For advice on coping with less acute eczema, see page 103.)

Hayfever is an allergy to pollens and other minute substances such as dust, animal hair and house mites. Often the condition naturally becomes worse during the summer months when there is a high level of pollen in the atmosphere.

SELF-HELP

- **Bach flower remedies** Keep calm by using Rescue Remedy, four drops as needed, especially if your problems are made worse by being stressed.

- **Aromatherapy** Essential oils can be used to help you relax – any oils which are known to be calming are suitable unless you are allergic to the pollen of a specific plant, eg lavender, camomile, orange blossom (neroli). However, eczema responds well to the addition of oils such as camomile and lavender to the bathwater, using each oil separately in a continuous cycle: one week of lavender, one week of camomile, and one week without either. Use four drops, diluted in 5ml/1 teaspoon of carrier oil.

- **Massage** Even if you are not able to use essential oils, you will benefit from regular massage throughout pregnancy to increase your sense of relaxation. If an asthmatic attack threatens, deep slow shoulder massage may be helpful in reducing the intensity of the attack.

- **Breathing exercises** SOS – Sigh Out Slowly– breathing (see page 66) and any assistance with regulating breathing patterns helps to reduce the length of an asthma attack. If you start to hyperventilate (over-breathe), whoever is with you should get you to focus on them, with eye-to-eye contact. They should then start breathing at the same rate as you, but very swiftly take control of the situation by forcibly slowing down their own breathing, while maintaining the eye-to-eye contact. You will find that you will automatically follow their lead and your own breathing will slow down and become more regular. (This is also a good technique to remember if you hyperventilate in labour.)

- **Nutritional therapy** Many people with eczema are deficient in zinc and essential fatty acids, including evening primrose oil (EPO). Supplements of both are in order unless you are also epileptic, when you should refrain from taking the EPO. A cream containing EPO can be applied to the skin. Your body's natural ability to utilize essential fatty acids from the foods you eat may be enhanced by reducing the amount of refined carbohydrates you consume – instead, eat wholegrain breads and cereals, brown rice and organic potatoes.
Hayfever sufferers may find their overall sensitivity to pollens and other triggers reduced by correcting food allergies, although this should not be attempted until after delivery of your baby as it involves excluding

foods in rotation from your diet in order to find out which are responsible for your allergies. However, you may be helped by increasing the vitamin C and magnesium content of your diet.

Asthma has many causes, but may be made worse by an allergy to wheat products, so try omitting these. In all cases, where possible avoid the artificial additives and preservatives added to processed foods.

OTHER THERAPIES WHICH MAY HELP

For these therapies, refer to a qualified practitioner.

Homeopathy is not suitable for self-medication here because the causes of these three conditions are so complex. However, homeopathy is probably one of the most effective therapies in the long term for any of these problems which persist once you have delivered.

Osteopathy or **chiropractic** can be beneficial during the postnatal period, in dealing with the ongoing effects and complications. These therapies may be useful during pregnancy, through realignment of the spine, in reducing the effects of any or all of the conditions.

Acupuncture to rebalance your energies can assist in preventing or reducing the frequency of asthmatic attacks, and may also help with relieving tensions or stimulating meridians to make you less susceptible to the substances that trigger eczema or hayfever.

Reflexology is relaxing, but can also stimulate production of your own steroid chemicals, which may help to reduce the severity of conditions such as eczema.

vaginal infections

Vaginal infections are relatively common in pregnancy due to changes which occur in the acidity of the vagina, plus an increase in mucus production. The most common infection is thrush, caused by a fungus, but bacteria, viruses or other organisms can lead to chlamydia, trichomonas or gonorrhoea. Most infections cause an irritating discharge which may be whitish, yellow or greenish and may have an unpleasant odour. Normal vaginal discharge is quite thick and white but should not cause irritation or smell particularly offensive. Sometimes the infection also causes urinary symptoms such as a burning sensation on passing urine or increased frequency; an unpleasant side effect of vaginal infection is soreness and perhaps pain on intercourse.

Many of these conditions will be transferred between you and your partner during sexual intercourse, so treatment of both partners is important to prevent continuing problems. If the infection is present in the vagina at the time of delivery, the baby can be affected as s/he travels down the birth canal and may then develop problems such as eye infections.

Medical treatment involves suppression of the symptoms and destruction of the organism causing the infection, but complementary medicine aims to look at the whole person and where possible tackle the factors which have made you more susceptible to the infection. Unfortunately, normal pregnancy changes are usually responsible for infections such as thrush, but steps can be taken to reduce the risks. It is worth noting that repeated courses of antibiotics can in themselves be responsible for persistent thrush and you would therefore be wise to challenge your family doctor if s/he is intent on prescribing additional courses of antibiotics (for any condition).

Another infection of the genitalia is herpes, caused by the same type of virus as triggers cold sores. This condition can initially make you seriously ill, but it is possible for the herpes virus to linger in your body after the acute illness has passed and for less serious recurrences to continue for some years.

When to seek further advice

Any vaginal discharge you are worried about should be reported to your family doctor, although not all discharges warrant medication. Any bleeding is, however, abnormal unless it is a very minor 'show' just before labour starts. If you become aware that you have herpes it must be treated before you go into labour to prevent it being passed to the baby, who may suffer long-term effects from it: if herpes has not gone into remission before labour commences you will probably be advised by your obstetrician to have a Caesarean section.

SELF-HELP

- **Nutritional therapy** Sugar and yeast products make you more susceptible to thrush, so try to eliminate these from your daily diet. Such products include beef extract, frozen or concentrated orange juice, cheese, bread made with yeast, alcohol, grapes and grape juice, raisins, sultanas, and B vitamins unless labelled as yeast-free.
  Garlic is a natural antifungal agent and the cloves can be eaten raw daily as a preventative measure. If thrush develops, a single clove of garlic, unpeeled to avoid stinging of the vaginal walls, well oiled and wrapped in muslin, can be inserted into the vagina and left for two to three hours. Zinc and iron tablets can be taken to correct any deficiencies which may have contributed to your susceptibility to vaginal infection and will help to boost your immune system.

- **Aromatherapy** Tea tree essential oil has been extremely well documented since as early as 1985 as an effective treatment for thrush and other vaginal infections, including severe and uncommon ones. Research into the effectiveness of tea tree oil for herpes and warts, including genital ones, is ongoing and gaining credibility among orthodox doctors. The even more effective, more recently discovered oils of kanuka and manuka from New Zealand can be used but may be difficult to find. Add two drops of oil to 250ml of boiled water, then dip a tampon in the water until it is soaked through; insert this into your vagina and replace it every two hours for two to three days. You will need to use a tampon which has an applicator so that the tampon does not expand before you attempt to insert it. Alternatively, you can dip a cotton wool ball in the tea tree solution and wipe it around the vaginal opening. Make sure that the solution is not too strong, as tea tree in itself can occasionally be an irritant, especially to the delicate vaginal lining. Proprietary tea tree pessaries are also available from healthfood stores.

- **Bach flower remedies** Crab apple can be used in your bath to reduce the feelings of uncleanliness you may have. If the irritation is making you emotionally irritable you could also take impatiens, two drops in water orally, three times a day.

- **Herbal remedies** Herbs which act on the immune system may be able to prevent further complications: try marigold, purple cone flower, thyme or wild indigo in combination with herbs which help to restore the mucous membranes such as golden rod, ground ivy or plantain. If herpes is present, herbs which are nerve tonics, such as vervain and lavender, may help, and dandelion or burdock will act as an internal cleanser and restorative.

● Live natural yogurt containing acidophilus (*not* fruit-flavoured from the local supermarket!) on a tampon is an effective method of relieving vaginal thrush.

Homeopathy

Take one 30C tablet of the most appropriate remedy three times daily for three days.

- If the discharge is offensive, profuse, brown or thick white like cottage cheese, causes itching and vaginal and vulval dryness or rawness; there is pain on intercourse and you have a desire to drink vinegar – sepia.
- If the discharge is thick white or yellow, profuse, burning, causes itching and is worse after exercising; you have an extreme thirst for large quantities of water – natrum mur.
- If the discharge is a creamy, slimy mucus, profuse, burning, causes itching and is worse when you become hot, but you have little thirst – pulsatilla.

hypertension (raised blood pressure)

Blood pressure is the force exerted by the blood on the walls of the blood vessels. Systolic pressure reflects the maximum pressure of blood against the walls of the arteries and is an indication of how strongly the left side of the heart is able to pump out the blood into the arteries. Diastolic pressure reflects the constant pressure on the artery walls and shows how resistant the blood vessel walls are. Blood pressure recordings are written with the systolic pressure over the diastolic pressure, but in pregnancy it is the diastolic pressure that is the more significant. There is a range of 'normal' blood pressure levels, but the diastolic will probably be between 60 and 80 and the systolic between 100 and 130.

Several changes occur in the circulation during pregnancy as a result of hormonal influences, increasing weight and the extra tissues required for the baby to develop and grow. If your blood pressure is taken in the first three months, it is likely to be the nearest to your normal non-pregnant level – this is called the baseline blood pressure. In the second three months, there is usually a fall in pressure due to relaxation of the blood vessel walls by the hormones, which causes the blood to flow through them more slowly and with less pressure. This is despite the increase in blood volume by about 25 per cent. As you approach the end of your pregnancy, your blood pressure may rise slightly because of the extra weight and other stresses, but should not normally increase by more than 20 above the baseline diastolic pressure of the first three months.

High blood pressure can occur during pregnancy either because you already had a problem (called essential hypertension) before conception, or as a result of the pregnancy – this is called gestational hypertension. If gestational hypertension is accompanied by swollen ankles and protein in your urine, it is called pre-eclampsia, which, if left untreated, can go on to become eclampsia, in which the mother has epileptic-type fits and the health of both mother and baby is compromised. True eclampsia is very rare (in more than 20 years as a midwife I have only known of a handful of cases), but pregnancy care aims to detect high blood pressure early enough to be able to treat it promptly and prevent further complications.

The women who are most at risk of developing any of these forms of hypertension include those whose pre-pregnancy blood pressure is high; mothers who are overweight or expecting more than one baby; diabetics; those who have a family or previous personal history of pregnancy hypertension; as well as women who are pregnant for the first time or with a new partner. Hypertension can interfere with the efficiency of the placenta, leading to poor growth and development and the birth of an immature and unwell baby.

Complementary therapies can be used to maintain a sense of well-being and relaxation to keep your blood pressure within manageable limits and occasionally to supplement the medical care required if it becomes too high.

When to seek further advice

In the early stages of pregnancy hypertension most women feel well, and it is only when the condition worsens that you begin to feel unwell. The swelling in your ankles may spread to your legs, hands, face and even your lower back. The other symptoms which you may experience in this situation relate to internal fluid retention: spots in front of your eyes and other visual disturbances occur because there is swelling around the nerves which serve the eyes; headaches – which, unlike early pregnancy ones, are usually at the front of your head – occur due to swelling generally around the brain; nausea and sickness result from fluid around the vomiting centre in the brain; pain underneath the right rib is a sign of fluid around the liver. If you develop any of these symptoms or feel in any way 'under the weather' you should contact your midwife or doctor, who can examine you more thoroughly.

SELF-HELP

- **Aromatherapy** A good deal of research has been conducted which demonstrates that several essential oils can have an effect on blood pressure. Certain oils are known to raise the pressure and should be avoided if you are at any risk of developing hypertension: these include rosemary, fennel, hyssop and sage. On the other hand, lavender, camomile, ylang ylang, neroli and rosewood have been shown to reduce blood pressure and aid relaxation. Trials on elderly people in nursing homes and on very ill people with heart problems in intensive care units have shown that lavender and neroli are particularly effective, and both are safe to use during pregnancy. Use four drops of essential oil, diluted in 5ml/1 teaspoon of carrier oil.
- **Massage** This can be extremely relaxing, too, and it has also been shown that it can have positive effects on people with hypertension. A pleasant back, neck, shoulder or foot massage induces a feeling of calm; if combined with essential oils as above, the effects may be even greater. Indeed, much research has focused on the question of whether the sedative effects of essential oils arise from the chemical constituents or as a result of the method of administration, ie massage.

- **Bach flower remedies** Rescue Remedy or impatiens will help you to control feelings of irritability which can exacerbate high blood pressure; if you are prone to tempers and rage, use cherry plum. If you are constantly 'on the go' and find it difficult to relax, try centaury.
- **Shiatsu** Self-administered shiatsu to the B2 points may help to maintain the blood pressure at reasonable levels (see fig. 3, page 208).
- **Tai Chi, Yoga** and **relaxation exercises** These can be beneficial if you already have a tendency towards high blood pressure, in order to prevent it becoming too high.
- **Nutritional therapy** Although controversial in relation to high blood pressure and pre-eclampsia, therapists specializing in nutrition advocate the use of vitamin and mineral supplements, in particular zinc and vitamin B6, as some trials have shown women with low levels of these nutrients to have an increased risk of the condition. Dealing with the effects of stress is important, too, as zinc is lost in the urine if you are stressed. A good multivitamin and mineral will also replace any deficiency in magnesium, calcium, and vitamins C and E. Nutrition experts have variously suggested through their trials that mothers who are vegan or very strongly vegetarian have less likelihood of developing pre-eclampsia, that reducing carbohydrate intake can improve the weight of the placenta and the baby, and that decreasing consumption of 'fast' foods, especially those with high levels of saturated fats, can also be beneficial. Without doubt, however, smoking has been shown to affect the health of the baby adversely if you develop pre-eclampsia and you should make every effort to cut down or stop smoking altogether.

Homeopathy

Take one 30C tablet of the most appropriate remedy three times daily for three days.

- If you have hypertension with swollen ankles but no protein in your urine (proteinuria); you feel better in the open air and emotionally feel shocked and fearful – opium.
- If you have hypertension with swollen ankles, feet, hands and fingers; you feel worse when cold and better when warm and lying down, and are anxious and find it difficult to concentrate – calcarea carbonica.

- If you have hypertension accompanied by proteinuria but no real swelling; you feel worse when sweating or passing urine and better after physical exertion; you are weary and you want to be left alone – gelsemium.
- If you have hypertension, swelling all over your body and proteinuria; you are intolerant to heat, irritable, fidgety, tearful and have a fear of death – apis.
- If you have hypertension, proteinuria, swelling and palpitations; you feel worse if cold and damp, after midnight, and are anxious and restless – arsenicum.
- If you have a sudden onset of the hypertension, swelling and proteinuria; you feel worse when touched and better when lying down; you have a throbbing sensation in your neck and are angry, confused and sensitive – belladonna.

Davina's story

Davina was referred to my complementary therapy clinic by her own community midwife because her blood pressure was slightly above normal limits when she was 32 weeks pregnant and it was thought that she would benefit from relaxation therapies. I suggested we try some reflexology and started to perform a visual and manual examination of her feet. As I worked on her toes, which represent the reflex zones for the eyes, I could feel irregularities under the skin which indicated some possible problems. Making an educated guess, I asked her how long she had had spots in front of her eyes, at which she burst into tears and queried how I knew. I told her that I had detected it from her feet and she informed me that when she had seen her midwife the day before she had lied when asked about any visual disturbances, because she had three other children at home and did not want to have to come into hospital. I then took her blood pressure, which was exceptionally high, and I immediately moved Davina to the delivery suite, where labour was induced and a tiny but fairly healthy baby boy was born, who was then transferred to the special care baby unit for routine observation.

OTHER THERAPIES WHICH MAY HELP

For these therapies, refer to a qualified practitioner.

Alexander technique can correct an habitually poor posture which may be causing tensions internally, contributing to the risk of raised blood pressure.

Chiropractic or **osteopathy** may realign the spine, eliminating or reducing stresses on the circulatory system.

Hypnotherapy could be appropriate where hypertension is made worse by severe stress and fear.

Reflexology can be used for general relaxation and reducing the blood pressure; the diagnostic potential of reflexology may assist in the identification of hidden symptoms indicating a worsening of your condition (see Davina's story).

vaginal bleeding

Miscarriage is the loss of a pregnancy before the twenty-fourth week when the baby is capable of living an independent existence. It occurs for many reasons, physical, hormonal or emotional, which may be due to your own health or that of the baby. About one in four pregnancies ends in miscarriage, often occurring even before the woman is aware she is pregnant; most happen within the first 12 weeks.

Miscarriage is a reaction of your body to some abnormality and seems to be nature's way of selecting the healthiest fertilized eggs to develop into live healthy babies. Sometimes you may experience a small amount of bleeding, which eventually stops – this is called a threatened miscarriage but fortunately the pregnancy continues safely. On other occasions, the bleeding continues and miscarriage becomes inevitable. Sometimes an inevitable miscarriage is complete and no further treatment is required, but more often blood clots and other debris, known as retained products of conception, need to be removed from your uterus under a general anaesthetic to ensure it is emptied fully and will work efficiently in the recovery phase.

Complementary therapies will not prevent a miscarriage that is meant to happen, but may assist in stopping the bleeding of a threatened miscarriage. They can also help you cope with the recovery phase following an inevitable miscarriage.

Bleeding which occurs after the twenty-fourth week of pregnancy is almost always abnormal (except for the slight loss which can occur temporarily following intercourse). The bleeding is either due to trauma and/or early partial separation of the placenta from the lining of the uterus, or to separation of a placenta which is lying abnormally low in the uterus. This means the placenta, which supplies oxygen and nutrients to the baby, is not fulfilling its function as well as it should.

When to seek further advice

If you start to bleed in early pregnancy you should consult your midwife or family doctor sooner rather than later. If miscarriage occurs and you continue to bleed heavily for more than a few days, *you should certainly seek help to prevent excessive haemorrhage.* In the event of bleeding in later pregnancy, *it is imperative that you consult your maternity care team and do not attempt to treat the condition yourself*, either by self-administration of natural remedies or by visiting a complementary practitioner who is not also a doctor or midwife. Supportive therapies can be used for relaxation when the bleeding slows down.

SELF-HELP

- **Nutritional therapy** This has a large part to play in ensuring that you are in good health before conception and in the early weeks of pregnancy, especially if you have had previous miscarriages. A diet rich in iron-containing foods such as dark green vegetables, red meats, whole grains, potatoes, eggs, nuts, dried fruits and seaweed will help to prevent severe anaemia even when bleeding is profuse; citrus fruits and juices assist the absorption of iron from these foods. A good multivitamin and mineral supplement containing vitamin B complex, zinc, magnesium, selenium and others is also useful. Consuming a clove of raw garlic daily will assist in preventing infection which can trigger miscarriage, as it is an extremely effective antiseptic.
- **Aromatherapy** It is best to avoid using essential oils in the first three months of pregnancy if you have a history of previous miscarriages, or in the current pregnancy while bleeding continues, as some of the chemical constituents in the oils may accelerate the process or increase bleeding after a miscarriage has occurred. However, they can be used for massage or added to the bathwater to help you recover physically

and emotionally afterwards – use a maximum of four drops of any of the suggested oils, diluted in 5ml/1 teaspoon of carrier oil, once daily. Ylang ylang, bergamot, neroli or lavender will be relaxing, and lavender, tea tree and naiouli help to prevent infection and aid healing. Melissa is wonderful for uplifting your spirits after a bereavement – one drop placed in the centre of the palm of your hand and sniffed has a good effect. However, make sure that you buy the best quality melissa to avoid oil which has been adulterated – but true melissa is very expensive. If you experience bleeding later in pregnancy it is again important to avoid using essential oils which are thought to trigger uterine contractions, but once the bleeding has slowed down or stopped you can use the oils for relaxation. Orange or camomile are both very gentle oils which can be added to the bath.

● **Bach flower remedies** Gentian could be useful if you feel generally depressed and despondent, sweet chestnut may lift feelings of total despair. Star of Bethlehem is helpful in many cases of bereavement; pine can be added if you have a tendency to blame yourself; willow if you feel full of resentment and keep asking 'Why me?'; and crab apple is appropriate if you feel generally unclean. If, later on, you are constantly putting on a 'brave face', you could try agrimony. Two drops each of any or all of these in a small glass of water should be taken three times daily until your feelings lift. Where you are unable to select more appropriate remedies, Rescue Remedy, using four drops as required, is a good panacea.

● **Breathing exercises** Using the SOS – Sigh Out Slowly – method (see page 66) can help to calm you when you are going through the physical and emotional trauma of an inevitable miscarriage, and the surgery that may follow to ensure that the uterus contains no further blood clots.

Homeopathy

Homeopathy provides a means of assisting the process of recovery following cessation of bleeding or actual miscarriage. Take one 100C tablet (if you can obtain them) or one 30C tablet of the most appropriate remedy, three times daily for three days.

▪ Arnica is the universal remedy for the physical and emotional 'battering' which you have taken either while bleeding is continuing to threaten the progress of your pregnancy, or once miscarriage has occurred.

- Early miscarriage with dark red, profuse bleeding, often associated with constipation, poor urinary output or in women with ovarian disease; where stinging pain starts out at the sides in the ovarian region and gradually moves to become contractions – apis.
- If the bleeding is brought on by fright, anger or stress, and is copious and continuous – aconite.
- If bleeding occurs before 12 weeks, is associated with anaemia and constipation, and causes intense pain in the buttocks, back and thighs – kali carb.

OTHER THERAPIES WHICH MAY HELP

For these therapies, refer to a qualified practitioner.

Herbal remedies may help. Crampbark is used for the relief of muscular tension and is a good remedy when the bleeding is known not to be due to hormonal disturbances. Chasteberry helps to balance hormones and may be used when bleeding occurs at around 8–12 weeks of pregnancy. This is usually given as a tincture, probably every half-hour to hour, until bleeding and any cramping pains have subsided. Raspberry leaf tea is useful for toning the uterus and may be prescribed by qualified herbalists for bleeding in early pregnancy. Lady's mantle or shepherd's purse are other herbs which can be effective.

Acupuncture can be used to rebalance your energies as, according to Traditional Chinese Medicine, your Yin–Yang balance may be disturbed. It may be possible to receive this treatment when bleeding has started in an attempt to prevent an inevitable miscarriage. If you have a history of previous miscarriages you could consult an acupuncturist before you subsequently attempt to conceive, so that your energy levels are in the optimum state to prevent further miscarriages.

Osteopathy or **chiropractic** could also be appropriate if you have suffered repeated miscarriages, as misalignments of the spine may be putting undue tensions on various organs, thereby disturbing hormonal output.

Alexander technique may also help, for the same reasons.

Reflexology is relaxing and will also assist in the expulsion of any clots from the uterus immediately following the miscarriage, but it is important that your reflexologist has a thorough understanding of the physiological processes

involved in miscarriage in order to prevent any unnecessary further bleeding.
Shiatsu or **massage** may engender a degree of emotional relaxation in the days and weeks following miscarriage.

Hypnotherapy might be appropriate in helping you to come to terms with the loss, especially if the grief is uncontrollable, perhaps after repeated miscarriages.

Jenny's story

Jenny came to see me for relief of various discomforts of pregnancy. She was delighted to be pregnant because she had already had three miscarriages following a long period of infertility. She told me, however, that she had been having osteopathic treatment during the past 12 months and that her osteopath had found that there was tension on the neck vertebrae in Jenny's spine. This, she was told, was putting undue stress on the pituitary gland in the brain, from which hormones that regulate the menstrual cycle and maintain pregnancy are produced. Four treatments by the osteopath to release the tension in her neck were sufficient for Jenny to conceive successfully – and by the time she came to see me she was already 23 weeks pregnant, so well past the time when miscarriage was likely to occur. Jenny went on to deliver a beautiful baby boy at 38 weeks of pregnancy.

multiple pregnancy

If you are expecting more than one baby, you are likely to be planning to give birth in hospital because, although the pregnancy may progress without problems, twin or triplet (or more) pregnancy is considered to be abnormal and warrants close medical supervision. This is mainly due to the increased risk of complications, and is usually a preventative measure. The potential difficulties which you may experience during pregnancy and labour include exacerbation of the normal physical discomforts of pregnancy, such as:

- Nausea and vomiting due to higher hormone levels.
- Heartburn and indigestion because of greater pressure.

- Swelling and varicose veins in your legs or vulva due to the extra weight burden.
- Tiredness, nightmares and insomnia as a result of being especially uncomfortable, your mind being over-active, and carrying more weight.
- Backache and sciatica due to the weight and hormones.

More serious complications may occur as a result of the increased weight, hormone levels and over-stretching of your uterus. These include high blood pressure, severe anaemia or haemorrhage, premature births or a slow or obstructed labour as a result of the position, size or health of the babies.

It is vital to prevent these complications or to detect them early enough to treat them before they become worse. Complementary therapies, therefore, should only be used to help you deal with the symptoms of the pregnancy, but nevertheless should always be used with the full knowledge of your doctor and midwife.

SELF-HELP

- **Nutritional therapy** A well-balanced diet is essential and you should try to consume adequate amounts of protein foods to provide the correct nourishment to enable your babies to grow. Follow the guidelines given on page 146. Giving up smoking is even more important than when you are expecting only one baby, because both (or all) your babies will already be smaller than one would be. You may wish to take a good quality multivitamin and mineral supplement, or zinc on its own.
- **Bach flower remedies** You will undoubtedly feel more anxious during this pregnancy than one where there is only one baby. Try aspen if you are fearful but not sure what you are frightened of. Elm may help if you feel overwhelmed by the responsibility of having two babies, or hornbeam if you are immensely weary at the thought of all the work you have to do – this is especially good once the babies are born. You will feel more than usually tired and may benefit from taking olive on a regular basis. Rock rose will help with nightmares and walnut will assist you in adapting to the major changes pending in your life (and your partner's!).

- **Homeopathy** Your body and mind will feel more than normally bruised and battered and you should use arnica following the delivery. If you are fortunate enough to have vaginal births of the babies, take one 30C tablet of arnica every two hours for three days, but if you have an operative delivery use arnica and hypericum, following the regime on page 117. If you suffer serious haemorrhage during or after the delivery of the placenta, take one 30C tablet of China every five minutes until it subsides.
- **Aromatherapy** Take care to use low doses (three to four drops of essential oil maximum) to avoid compromising the babies' health, particularly during labour. Citrus oils plus ylang ylang or sandalwood are safe oils; it is best to avoid geranium near the time of the birth, as it may interfere with the clotting mechanisms in your blood and trigger more severe haemorrhage. You should avoid using those oils which are thought to trigger uterine contractions, because of the risk of early labour. These are the same oils that are used for pain relief in labour (see Pain and discomfort in labour, page 158).
- **Hydrotherapy** Walking and movement become very difficult towards the end of pregnancy when you are expecting more than one baby, but relaxing or exercising gently in water improves mobility due to the buoyancy, and can also enhance your confidence and self-esteem.

OTHER THERAPIES WHICH MAY HELP

For these therapies, refer to a qualified practitioner.

Osteopathy or **chiropractic** can help relieve your discomforts. As backache, sciatica and symphysis pubis (pubic bone) pain can be much more distressing because of the increased weight which puts an extra curvature into your spine, you would benefit from ongoing treatment. This would relieve some of the physical discomforts, but will also realign your skeleton following delivery, as the after-effects of pregnancy and birth can persist for up to a year.

Homeopathy is more difficult to self-prescribe in a multiple pregnancy, as many of the relatively minor discomforts of pregnancy can become so much more serious if you are expecting more than one baby. You would be wise, therefore, to consult a practitioner who can identify the full symptom picture to ensure the most appropriate solution from the beginning.

5

the birth

Labour and delivery are the culmination of the nine months of waiting: the end of the beginning. You will have spent many months wondering – and probably worrying – about how you will cope during the labour; sometimes it will have been difficult to see beyond this time and to imagine how you will be affected by your new arrival, especially if this is your first baby.

Conventional antenatal care aims to prepare you physically and mentally for the birth and parenthood but, with so many expectant mothers to care for, it can be almost impossible to fulfil the needs of every individual. If you have questions, concerns or worries, your midwife or obstetrician will be glad to discuss them with you, but you may have to initiate the conversation.

There are many excellent groups and classes which offer you opportunities to prepare for the birth, and numerous books are to be found in libraries and shops. However, there are also many ways in which you can help to maintain your health during pregnancy, prepare yourself for the birth, and deal with the discomforts of labour by using complementary therapies.

well-being during pregnancy

You will want to be in the best possible health during pregnancy while your baby is developing and growing, and in readiness for the arduous task of labour. Well-being is about feeling good – physically, emotionally and spiritually – and you will have many issues to consider that are outside the scope of this book. However, if you make every effort to ensure optimum physical health and emotional well-being, many of the other issues, including spiritual ones, will fall into perspective.

When to seek further advice

Your midwife, family doctor and obstetrician are available to monitor your progress during pregnancy, labour and after the birth, to prepare you for delivery and new parenthood, and to detect early and treat promptly any complications that arise. If at any time you feel unwell or are unsure as to whether or not something is normal, do not hesitate to ask their advice, so that they can help you to cope with your pregnancy and enjoy it as much as you are able. If you think that your baby's movement pattern has changed from what you consider to be normal, ask your midwife to examine you and listen to the baby's heartbeat. If you have *any vaginal bleeding at all* check it out with your midwife or doctor. All the professionals involved in your care want you to achieve a safe and satisfying delivery of your new baby with as few complications as possible.

SELF-HELP

- **Nutritional therapy** Eat as well balanced a diet as possible. Include at least five portions of fruit and vegetables daily and preferably 3 litres of water. Try to avoid too many artificial additives in the food you buy – look out for these in processed and preserved foods – as well as coffee, tea, cola and alcohol. High consumption of caffeine has been associated with babies being small and ill at birth, so you should try where possible to restrict the number of cups of coffee to less than three a day. Eat reasonable amounts of unrefined carbohydrates, including wholewheat breads, cereals, pastas, and some first- or second-class proteins such as meat, poultry, fish, beans and other legumes. Eating plenty of sea fish increases the weight and health of your baby and may prevent pre-term labour. Avoid eating too many foods which contain high quantities of fats such as full-fat cheeses, fried foods or fatty meats. Reduce your intake of sugar and salt where feasible.

  You might like to consider the addition of a good quality multivitamin and mineral supplement, especially if you have recently been on the contraceptive Pill, live in a very urbanized area or partake of noxious substances such as alcohol, cigarettes or drugs, including those necessary for any pre-existing medical condition. If you are very stressed, zinc is lost in your urine and you are less able to absorb it from the foods you eat, so you may consider taking a zinc supplement.

- **Bach flower remedies** Panic attacks are extremely common during pregnancy, for many reasons, but Rescue Remedy can be a means of relieving them. If you are frightened about the birth try mimulus or larch. Vivid dreams, sometimes remembered as nightmares, are also common as you progress towards the end of pregnancy. If you wake up suddenly in the middle of the night, Rescue Remedy can be used again, or if you need to 'switch off' your mind before settling to sleep, try white chestnut.

- **Yoga, Tai Chi** or **relaxation exercises** Any of these forms of exercise will encourage suppleness and fitness in preparation for the birth, as well as inducing a sense of relaxation and calm. They may also help in the relief of some of the physical discomforts of pregnancy (see Chapter 3).

- **Hydrotherapy** In the form of gentle swimming or specific antenatal exercise in water, this will assist with mobility, ease aches and pains, and reduce oedema. On a psychological level, this type of exercise engenders a greater sense of self-esteem than you may otherwise have, as a result of your increasing size and changing shape. The therapeutic effects of water can also be obtained by using a foot bath in which to relax your feet, with essential oils added if you wish.

- **Massage** If you can ask someone to massage you regularly during your pregnancy this can be very effective in keeping you relaxed, both physically and mentally. Regular full body massage throughout pregnancy will have a cumulative effect, which may be felt during labour. It is possible to perform self-massage for specific problems, but the relaxation effects are not so marked. However, you may wish to perform massage of the perineum (the area between the lower edge of your vagina and the anus), as this has been found to help the area stretch more easily during labour in order to enlarge the birth opening, and possibly to prevent tearing or the need for an episiotomy (cut). Perineal massage is best performed while you are in the bath or lying on your bed. A small amount of almond or olive oil can be used for lubrication. Insert the thumb of your dominant hand into your vaginal opening with your second and third fingers on the outside. Gently massage the perineal area between your thumb and fingers, using an upwards and outwards movement, for about five minutes a day from approximately 35 weeks of pregnancy.

- **Aromatherapy** Keep calm and relaxed by adding essential oils such as camomile, lavender, ylang ylang, bergamot or geranium to your bathwater – mix four drops with 5ml/1 teaspoon of carrier oil. Use several oils in succession so that you do not continue to use the same oil for more than three weeks.

- **Herbal remedies** Raspberry leaf tea is a good uterine toner. You can start to drink it from about 28 weeks of pregnancy, commencing with one cup daily for two to three weeks, to allow your body to become accustomed to it; then increase to two cups daily for two to three weeks; then finally, from about 36 weeks, take three cups a day – one in the morning, one at midday and one at night. You should, however, refrain from using raspberry leaf if you have a history of pre-term labour, have had a Caesarean section, or have had more than four children, and if in this pregnancy you have been admitted to hospital for pre-term labour contractions or are carrying more than one baby, as your uterus will be more sensitive to its effects.

- **Pelvic floor exercises** During labour your pelvic floor muscles, which form a hammock-shaped area between the openings to your vagina and your rectum, will be stretched to facilitate the birth of your baby. This can be likened to a piece of elastic – if the muscles are over-stretched during labour they become slack and will not tighten up again. You will be actively encouraged to practise pelvic floor exercises (sometimes called kegel exercises) following the birth of your baby, but you can assist this process by starting before delivery. Imagine the squeezing movement that you do when trying to stop yourself from passing urine, or perhaps to increase sensation during sexual intercourse. It is this same movement which is the basis of the exercises – you should aim to hold each muscle contraction for up to ten seconds before releasing and repeating ten times. However, you should not practise the exercise while you are actually passing urine – although this is a means of testing how effective the exercises are, repeatedly clenching your muscles during the passage of urine will cause a minor backwards flow of urine that can trigger urinary tract infections. (See also Massage, page 147.)

OTHER THERAPIES WHICH MAY HELP

For these therapies, refer to a qualified practitioner.

Reflexology or **shiatsu** is very relaxing and may also treat specific ailments. Research by one family doctor found that women who had regular reflexology during pregnancy experienced labours which were less painful, shorter and with fewer complications than those of women who had not had the treatment.

Alexander technique can re-educate your posture, helping to ease backache and other symptoms of pregnancy. Some of the exercises you may be encouraged to perform, such as squatting, help to prepare you for various positions which may be required in labour.

Acupuncture can remedy any imbalance in the energies flowing along the meridians that is caused by anxiety about labour, as well as relieving physical discomforts of pregnancy. Research trials have found that if acupuncture is received regularly during pregnancy it may shorten the duration of labour by up to two hours in mothers having their first babies, yet other trials have found the length of labour increased, although good pain relief was achieved! Acupuncture may also be of help during pregnancy for giving up smoking.

Osteopathy is generally seen as a therapy that is appropriate if you have a bad back or other tangible problem. However, an osteopath is also able to assist in the maintenance of your well-being during pregnancy by reducing the impact of the physical effects caused by hormones or your increasing weight.

Cranial osteopathy, a subsidiary of osteopathy, is extremely relaxing and can be used to correct physical discomforts and emotional dis-ease, although of course it will not deal with the causes of any stress.

Chiropractic used for back pain in pregnancy has been shown to reduce the incidence of similar pain during labour by 84 per cent, while other research has shown that chiropractic during pregnancy can reduce the length of the first stage of labour by almost half, both in women having their first baby and those experiencing subsequent pregnancies.

Hypnotherapy can be helpful if you are very anxious about any special tests and investigations, or if a previous pregnancy unfortunately ended in miscarriage or stillbirth, or if you have a history of pre-term labour. It can also help with giving up smoking. If you are considering using hypnotherapy for pain relief in labour, you should consult a therapist early enough in pregnancy to enable you to practise the techniques you will be taught.

breech presentation

During the early months of pregnancy while the baby is still growing, s/he is able to move around freely in the bag of fluid within the uterus. However, towards the end of the pregnancy most babies will settle into a head-first (cephalic) presentation, as this is the most favourable position for delivery. The baby's head is the largest part which must negotiate the mother's bony pelvic canal, and once the head is delivered s/he starts to breathe even before the rest of the body emerges. During the first stage of labour the head also presses down on the cervix (neck of the uterus), facilitating dilation in readiness for the birth itself.

A small number of babies, however, settle into a bottom-first, or breech presentation. This could be for many reasons: a big baby in a relatively small pelvis; an obstruction in the lowest part of the uterus such as an abnormally low placenta or fibroids; a funnel-shaped pelvis; or twins, where one baby is cephalic and the other breech. Whatever the reason, a breech birth is not considered normal and does carry some risks to both mother and baby. The usual management today is to offer you a Caesarean section so that the birth can be controlled and the risk of problems minimized, although you do have every right to challenge this proposal.

A few obstetricians are now returning to the procedure of external cephalic version in which they attempt, by manipulation of your abdomen, to encourage your baby to turn to head-first. This approach was very popular about 20 years ago and obstetricians were experienced and therefore very successful with the procedure. It went out of fashion for many years, but has recently been resurrected as one way of avoiding Caesarean section, although lack of experience among contemporary obstetricians means that it is not always successful. Here are a few suggestions for trying complementary therapies which may be more successful in preventing you having a Caesarean section for breech presentation.

SELF-HELP

- **Yoga** Some authorities have shown that assuming the all-fours position – with your forearms flat on the ground and your bottom higher than your head – for 20 minutes a day from about 32 weeks of pregnancy, can encourage a breech baby to turn to head-first. It is simple and therefore worth trying, but is rather uncomfortable for a prolonged period of time. This technique can be combined with reflexology or moxibustion (see opposite).
- **Homeopathy** A single high dose of pulsatilla (200C if possible) can work in some cases of breech presentation, especially if this remedy is considered to be your constitutional remedy: that is, the one which best matches your personality type.
- **Herbal remedies** Building on the use of the Bl67 acupuncture point

(see Moxibustion, below) a paste of fresh ginger can be applied to the little toes before going to bed, in order to turn the baby from breech to head-first. This is a part of Traditional Chinese Medicine and the ginger acts as a heat source over the Bl67 point in much the same way as the moxa sticks. In one study, over a hundred women at between 28 and 32 weeks of pregnancy applied this treatment, compared to a group of over two hundred women with breech presentation who had no treatment. After only one treatment almost 50 per cent of the babies had turned and after several treatments, almost 75 per cent were head-first, compared to about 50 per cent in the untreated group.

OTHER THERAPIES WHICH MAY HELP

For these therapies, refer to a qualified practitioner.

Hypnotherapy may be of help. A trial undertaken in the mid-1990s divided women with breech presentations into two groups: one to receive hypnotherapy, the other to have no treatment. Hypnosis included asking the mothers to explain why they thought their babies were in the breech position. Women with breech babies often report feeling that their lives are upside down, and it is thought that there is an emotional as well as a physical element related to the baby's position. The number of babies in the hypnosis group who turned from breech to head-first was twice that of the babies in the no-treatment group.

Reflexology, sometimes combined with **acupressure** working on the Bl67 point, can be effective in some women.

Moxibustion to turn a breech baby

Moxibustion is part of Traditional Chinese Medicine (see Acupuncture, page 28), in which moxa sticks are used as a heat source over the relevant acupuncture points. Moxa sticks are rolled, compressed, dried mugwort, a herb. The ends of two sticks are lit and the flames are quenched, leaving a smoking, glowing tip, like an incense stick but bigger. The smoking tips are held over the Bl67 acupuncture points at the base of the nail of the little toes of each foot (see fig. 4, page 209), a couple of centimetres away from the skin so that there is a sensation of warmth but it is not unbearably hot. The treatment is carried out for 15 minutes twice a day for up to five days, at around 33–34 weeks of pregnancy, although it can be done at any time up to the end of pregnancy. Usually the midwife or acupuncturist will show you how to do the first treatment and then send you home to carry on by yourself.

Moxibustion is thought to work by stimulating both the heart rate and movements of the baby, and the sensitivity and contractility of the uterus so that the muscle layer becomes irritable and responsive to changes in the baby's position (but it will not trigger labour prematurely).

In order to be eligible for the treatment, it is important that you do not have any uterine scars from previous operations, are between 33 and 40 weeks pregnant with only one baby, have had no bleeding, placental separation or excess fluid surrounding the baby during the pregnancy, and no complications such as high blood pressure, diabetes or heart disease. It is vital that the position of the baby is checked before you start the treatment in case s/he has already turned.

Many obstetricians dismiss the value of trying moxibustion, claiming that many babies will turn themselves if left for long enough, which is true. However, a very large research trial in China in 1998, conducted by Italian doctors, divided expectant mothers with breech presentation into three groups: one group was left alone (control group); one group was offered external cephalic version; and one group was given moxibustion. Despite the fact that some babies in each group turned spontaneously to a cephalic presentation, the number of normal, head-first, vaginal deliveries at around 40 weeks of pregnancy was greatest in the group of mothers who had used the moxibustion.

If you wish to try moxibustion to turn your baby from breech to head-first, you will need to find either an acupuncturist who specializes in caring for pregnant women or a midwife who has been trained to undertake the procedure.

Sam's story

Sam already had three children from her previous marriage but was now expecting her first baby with her new partner. She came to see me when she was 35 weeks pregnant and her baby was in the breech position. She was eager to try moxibustion in order to avoid a Caesarean section, and I showed her how to do the procedure. She went home and used the moxa sticks twice a day over the next three days. On the third day she was applying the heat to her feet with her children and partner watching, when everyone was amazed to see her abdomen suddenly start to heave and move about – she said it felt 'like an earthquake!' The next day she was due to have an appointment at the hospital with the obstetrician, who carried out an ultrasound scan to check the baby's position. He was quite surprised to find that the baby had, indeed, turned to a cephalic presentation – and was even more astounded when Sam told him how it had been achieved! Sam went on to have a beautiful baby girl at 38 weeks of pregnancy – a nice, normal, head-first delivery.

onset of labour

Normal pregnancy lasts for anything from 37 to 43 weeks and you can safely go into labour at any time during this period. You may have been given a specific date for your expected delivery, but this is only an estimate and should never be taken as an absolute. In some countries pregnant women are told they will have their babies some time within a four-week period, so that there is no heavy reliance on a specified date. There are many 'old wives' tales' regarding the beginning of labour and it is not true that first babies are always late or that girls trigger labour earlier than boys.

Several factors contribute to labour starting. Your uterus will only stretch so far, and when it reaches its maximum the uterine nerves become irritable and contractions commence: this is why women expecting very large babies or more than one baby often go into pre-term labour before 37 weeks of pregnancy (see page 170). Several hormone changes also occur, so that there is a fall in the levels of those responsible for maintaining the pregnancy, and a rise in other hormones which trigger contractions. Your baby plays a part in the process of labour, too, producing his/her own chemicals from the brain and the adrenal glands above the kidneys, which help to initiate labour. Towards the end of pregnancy the baby settles into a position which is usually the most favourable for delivery, and this helps to put pressure on the cervix (neck of the uterus) to start the process of opening up, or dilating.

Going into labour is a natural physiological event and should not be tampered with unless there is a medical justification for so doing. It is not wise to request labour to be induced (artificially started) either by conventional means or complementary therapies just because you are fed up with being pregnant, for once the process has been interfered with it is more likely to lead to the need for further intervention.

However, there are occasions when pregnancy is prolonged beyond the usually quoted 40 weeks and obstetricians may start to try to persuade you to have labour artificially induced. There are varying opinions about when induction should be carried out, which will depend on the knowledge, expertise and previous experience of the individual obstetrician, but this may range from ten days 'overdue' to three weeks, so long as the condition of mother and baby remains satisfactory. A friend of mine, who was booked to have her baby at home and went three-and-a-half weeks overdue, tried everything from eating curries to going on the 'big wheel' at the fair, but without success, and eventually she had to succumb to a hospital induction of labour!

You may like to utilize some complementary strategies to encourage a more natural onset of labour. Many suggestions will be made by other women, some based on fact and others being complete fiction. Here are my recommendations, most of which build on the body's own near-readiness to go into labour.

When to seek further advice

If anything occurs as you reach the end of pregnancy that causes you to worry, do consult your midwife. This includes vaginal bleeding, severe headaches, major changes in the baby's movement pattern or anything else about which you are unsure.

SELF-HELP

- **Massage** Massaging your nipples stimulates the production of the hormone oxytocin, which is responsible both for uterine contractions and for lactation. If you gently rub your nipples between forefinger and thumb, for about five minutes each day, you will increase the oxytocin levels and so stimulate uterine action. It is important to massage only one breast at a time, as doing both together can sometimes cause unnaturally strong contractions which squeeze the baby and temporarily reduce the supply of oxygen. While this occurs normally during labour contractions, it is not a good idea to encourage excessively strong contractions, especially before labour is well established.

- **Sexual intercourse** If you can summon up the energy to indulge in some pre-labour sex, it has been found to have a beneficial effect on inducing labour. This is because stimulation of the cervix by the penis causes a local release of prostaglandin, which is one of the hormones responsible for triggering labour, from just inside the cervix. Male semen also contains prostaglandin. Furthermore, if you achieve orgasm, this in itself causes mild uterine contractions which may, at this time, be sufficient to start labour.

- **Herbal remedies** If you have not already been drinking raspberry leaf tea (see Well-being during pregnancy, page 147) it is still not too late to start. Sip two to three cups a day to tone the uterus; the tea can also be taken during labour to facilitate uterine action.

- **Aromatherapy** Add four drops in total of lavender and clary sage, diluted in 5ml/1 teaspoon of carrier oil, to your bath and relax in it: these oils have been shown to have an effect on uterine action, while the relaxation may be sufficient to enable you mentally to 'let go' and start labour. An additional drop of jasmine can also help, but it must be of good quality to ensure that it has not been adulterated with another, cheaper oil.

- **Shiatsu** Intermittent pressure can be applied about 20–30 times to the acupuncture points which can stimulate labour: these are the Li4 points on the hands; the Bl67 points on the little toes; the GB21 points on the shoulders; and the sacral points B27–31 (see figs 1, 4 and 5, pages 208–9). The easiest points to stimulate yourself are the Li4 points on the webbing between the thumb and forefinger of each hand, while a more effective treatment can be performed by a qualified shiatsu practitioner on all the relevant points.

Homeopathy

Many people advocate the use of a specific homeopathic remedy – caulophyllum – for starting labour. However, this should not be taken simply because you are overdue, unless you match the symptom picture described below. Inappropriate use can lead to either a delay in establishing labour or excessively strong contractions, especially if you have a history of quick, easy labours.

A single dose of caulophyllum in the 30C potency can be used if you are past your due date, fretful and irritable, weak and exhausted. You may feel slightly nauseous and trembling, and be very thirsty. Any contractions you may experience will be weak, short, irregular, intermittent yet distressing and will feel as if they are flying about in all directions from your uterus to your bladder, groin and down your legs. Eventually they may cease completely because you are so exhausted. You will feel worse if you are cold but better if cool fresh air is circulating around you. There will be a profuse secretion of vaginal mucus and you may feel needle-like pains in the cervix.

Harriet's story

Harriet had been coming to my complementary therapy clinic for some weeks for treatment of several physical discomforts. I had been using reflexology, and from my examination of her feet at 39 weeks of pregnancy it seemed unlikely that she would go into labour within the next week. I suggested that Harriet continue to take her raspberry leaf tea, which she had commenced at 35 weeks, and that she should telephone me if she went overdue. I was not surprised to receive her call two weeks later when she had passed her due date, desperate to avoid an induction of labour. Her own midwife had already carried out an internal examination and a 'membrane sweep', which can sometimes speed up the onset of labour. I performed reflexology to the parts of the feet representing the uterus and the pituitary gland from which the labour hormones are produced, and incorporated acupressure to the Bl67 points on the little toes. I massaged Harriet's feet with a blend of essential oils including jasmine, nutmeg, clary sage and lavender. I then applied acupressure to the Li4 points on the hands, the GB21 points on the shoulders and the sacral points at the base of the spine. That same night she went into labour and gave birth to a lovely baby boy.

OTHER THERAPIES WHICH MAY HELP

For these therapies, refer to a qualified practitioner.

Reflexology, stimulating the foot zones for the uterus and the pituitary gland (see fig. 4, page 209) may be sufficient to initiate contractions. In my experience, these zones are a good indicator of whether or not labour is imminent. The exact reflexology points for the pituitary gland – the area in the brain from which pregnancy and labour hormones are produced – are on the backs of the big toes. The right toe relates to the front part of the pituitary gland, which produces hormones to maintain the pregnancy, and this part of the toe is tender throughout pregnancy; the pituitary zone on the left foot relates to the posterior part, which produces labour hormones in increasing amounts as pregnancy progresses. When these two very precise points are equal in tenderness, or the left is more tender, labour is imminent. I am able to predict from a pregnant mother's feet, with reasonable accuracy, when she will go into labour.

Shiatsu for a qualified practitioner to apply appropriate techniques to stimulate the onset of labour.

Acupuncture needles may be used on the same points as those worked by a shiatsu practitioner.

Homeopathy for a full assessment by a qualified therapist, followed by the prescription of remedies in addition to or instead of caulophyllum.

pain and discomfort in labour

Labour, the process of dilating the cervix and pushing the baby downwards so that s/he is ready to travel down the birth canal to be born, is – as the word suggests – hard work. It is also almost always painful due to the effects of muscle contractions in the uterus, the transmission of sensations along nerve endings to the brain and the impact of chemicals in the brain. The process of labour provides a mental opportunity to make the transition from being pregnant to being a mother, and indeed, those few women who 'escape' with a pain-free labour quite often feel as if they have missed out!

Pain is influenced by personal perception but may also be affected by various other factors, both positive and negative. Ensuring you are as fit and healthy as possible before labour, keeping well informed and being assertive enough to engage in a partnership with your midwife and doctor can all contribute positively to a reduction in your pain and discomfort during labour. Keeping upright and mobile helps your body, particularly your uterus, to do its work efficiently. Changing position, staying cool (emotionally as well as physically) and being accompanied by a birth companion of your choice will also contribute to a more positive and productive labour and delivery, so that you have a safe and satisfying experience with as little trauma to you or your baby as possible.

When to seek further advice

If your labour is long and drawn out or if you develop complications, your *perception* of the pain may make it feel much worse, especially if you are also anxious and frightened. There are, of course, various medical methods of pain relief for labour such as gas and oxygen, injections or epidural (spinal) anaesthesia. Do not feel a 'failure' if you can no longer cope with the pain of contractions, but ask for something more to help you. It is far better that you are assisted with coping with the pain so that labour remains as near normal as possible – trying to 'soldier on' with unbearable pain can sometimes lead to other complications.

SELF-HELP

- **Nutritional therapy** Eat small, frequent meals of carbohydrate foods such as toast, cereals and porridge which will give you energy. Ensure you drink plenty of fluids, as it is easy to become dehydrated once your body is working hard, especially if you are in hospital where the rooms are likely to be hot. It is not necessary to refrain from eating and drinking in labour unless you are due to have a Caesarean section.
- **Relaxation techniques** Remember to use your muscle relaxation technique and SOS – Sigh Out Slowly – breathing during each contraction (see page 66).
- **Aromatherapy** Essential oils can be used to good effect in labour, with certain oils thought to aid pain relief and others to facilitate

uterine action. Choose a blend of oils such as lavender, clary sage and a good quality jasmine – a maximum of four drops in total (including only one drop of jasmine), diluted in 5ml/1 teaspoon of carrier oil, is sufficient strength. The oils can be massaged into your shoulders, abdomen, feet or back, or they can be added to the bathwater as long as your waters have not broken, as this gives direct access to the baby's eyes via the vagina and cervix.

Peppermint or spearmint essential oils can be added, one drop neat, to a cottonwool ball and sniffed to combat nausea and sickness, and one drop of melissa, of good quality, can be put into the centre of the palm of your hand to inhale when you are feeling tired and emotional towards the end of labour.

If you wish to use oils in a vaporizer, you will need to check with the staff caring for you to ensure this is acceptable. Electrical vaporizers will need to be checked for wiring safety, so it is better if you have alerted the staff to your wishes before you actually arrive at the hospital in labour. If you are at home you could use two drops of oil (a single oil, or one drop each of two oils, of your choice) in a burner, but you will not be allowed to use this in hospital because of fire regulations. Any form of vaporized oil should be used intermittently (for about ten minutes in each hour) to avoid over-saturating the nostrils and causing nausea – not only for the sake of you and your birth companion but also for the staff!

You may be lucky enough to have your baby in an area where essential oils are used by the midwives as a normal part of labour care. The largest clinical aromatherapy trial in Europe was completed in 1998 at the John Radcliffe Hospital in Oxford, where over 8,000 mothers during a period of nine years were offered aromatherapy in labour. The results were extremely promising and showed that fewer drugs were used for pain relief (which was much cheaper for the unit), the length of many women's labours was reduced, and other symptoms such as sickness in labour could be treated. There was less than 1 per cent of adverse effects on women from the oils: these were minor, such as skin irritation, and none of the side effects occurred in the babies.

● **Massage** This can be wonderfully soothing, but you will need to wait until you are in labour to know whether or not you wish to be touched.

Some women want to be nurtured and 'mothered' while others wish to be left alone, in much the same way as a cat having kittens. Massage to the small of your back can relieve the back pain which accompanies certain positions of the baby, such as when the head is facing backwards. Foot massage can be very comforting and warming – labouring women quite literally suffer from 'cold feet', as the majority of the blood is directed away to those parts of the body involved in the exertion of labour. Shoulder massage can ease the tension caused by being in unnatural positions, especially at the time of the birth itself. Very light abdominal massage in a clockwise circular movement may influence your perception of the pain of uterine contractions, as touch impulses reach the brain before pain impulses.

- **Hydrotherapy** The use of water for labour and occasionally for the birth itself is well documented as having a beneficial effect on both the progress and pain of contractions. Relaxing in a bath of warm water which covers your abdomen will calm you and help you to cope with the contractions; research has also found that this makes the uterus work more efficiently so that the length of labour is reduced. Some women like to remain in the bath for the delivery, although you will be asked to get out of the water once the baby has been born and before the expulsion of the placenta so that any potential haemorrhage can be dealt with promptly. If you are planning a water delivery you should discuss this with your midwife early in your pregnancy so that the necessary arrangements can be made.

- **Shiatsu** You can ask your companion to perform a few shiatsu techniques during each contraction. The points are B27–31 (see fig. 5, page 209). Acupressure to the P6 point (see fig. 1, page 208) can also be used to relieve the nausea and vomiting that sometimes occurs in late labour.

- **Bach flower remedies** Rescue Remedy can be added to a small glass of water and sipped throughout labour to reduce general stress. Olive is useful if your labour is very long and you become tired. White chestnut is appropriate if you are constantly worried during the labour and cannot rid yourself of unwanted fears, while mimulus is a general remedy for fear when you are unsure of the cause. Willow can be used if you become self-pitying and introspective. Use two drops of each as required.

- **Herbal remedies** Raspberry leaf tea can be sipped throughout labour, either hot or iced, to facilitate uterine action. Ginseng may help to increase your energy and performance during a long, hard labour – there is considerable research to support this, but ginseng should be avoided if you have headaches or high blood pressure. It is not wise, either, to take it continually during pregnancy. Motherwort, as its name suggests, is good for labour, especially when it is slow to start or there are false starts, and skullcap helps to ease pain and disperse tensions which accompany the pain.

Homeopathy

Take one 30C tablet of the most appropriate remedy every 15 minutes, as required.

- For very frequent, painful contractions with soreness in your back, accompanied by a headache and fear that the baby will die; you feel worse if there is a lot of noise around you, even music – aconite.
- For distressing, irregular, spasmodic contractions which cause your uterus to become 'tired'; you are restless, cold and feel sore all over but fail to let people know how much you are suffering; despite this you feel better if someone is able to touch and 'mother' you – arnica.
- For unbearable, spasmodic contractions which shoot down your legs and labour is very long and apparently unproductive; typically you will say that you 'can't bear it any more'; you are rude, moan and toss about a lot causing perspiration, thirst and nausea; you are sensitive to noise and pain but feel better if you can be in fresh air – chamomilla.
- For short, irregular, ineffective contractions which are sharp and cramping and fly in all directions; if the cervix fails to dilate and you have a lot of mucus; you are fretful, exhausted, hot, thirsty and irritable, often trembling and feeling faint and nauseous – caulophyllum.
- For distressing, irregular and ineffective contractions which are cutting, especially in your back, coming on suddenly but easing off only gradually; your moods are changeable and you are apologetic, wanting sympathy and very distressed; pain relief is often sought spontaneously by pressing against the end of the bed with your feet – pulsatilla.
- For spasmodic contractions which shoot upwards; labour is often short and

sharp but you are weepy, anxious, restless and dictatorial with your eyes half-closed; you may be unable to pass urine adequately to empty your bladder and may develop flatulence; pain relief is often sought spontaneously by alternately pressing your feet against the end of the bed and then releasing – lycopodium.

OTHER THERAPIES WHICH MAY HELP

For these therapies, refer to a qualified practitioner.

Acupuncture has been well researched and in some countries, including Sweden and France, has been used for pain relief in labour since the 1970s. Sometimes acupuncture needles are inserted into the ear (auricular acupuncture), which has a complete set of acupuncture points in miniature – this helps you to remain mobile. Maternity units in some countries now offer an acupuncture-midwifery service, although this is not widespread and you may have to arrange to be accompanied in labour by an independent therapist. However, there is much more acceptance of acupuncture for pain relief these days and this should not cause a problem on condition that you inform your midwife and doctor well in advance. I remember meeting a lady when I was a community midwife in 1980, at a time when complementary medicine was less well accepted than it is today. She was so delighted that she had achieved the birth of her first baby at home with the help of acupuncture for pain relief that she proceeded to telephone all the local family docotrs to inform them of her success.

Reflexology will not only be relaxing but certain aspects can also help with the relief of pain, as well as facilitating uterine action where appropriate.

Hypnotherapy can be given by a hypnotherapist accompanying you during labour, although it is common practice and just as effective to consult the therapist during pregnancy. You will be taught how to hypnotize yourself, using a trigger or cue to induce the sense of relaxation and sedation.

Geraldine's story

I was privileged to look after Geraldine during the birth of her second baby. She had been attending my complementary therapy clinic for treatment of a range of physical symptoms and was due to have her last appointment with me. When she arrived she was in the early stages of labour, which seemed to have commenced during the night.

I took Geraldine through to the delivery suite and it was obvious that labour was progressing fast. A midwife whom she had met before was allocated to care for her. I said that I was able to stay with her for a short while, but that I had to attend a meeting at 12.30 (it was then 10.45). She was, however, in reasonable discomfort so I performed shiatsu and reflexology techniques during her contractions. Towards the end of the first stage of labour Geraldine became very weepy and distressed but also kept telling me what I should be doing, which was a marked change in her character. She seemed irritated by the noises of staff coming in and out of the room and I noticed her alternately pressing and relaxing her feet against the end of the bed, a sure indication for homeopathic lycopodium, which I gave her in a 30C strength. I also offered her some Bach flower Rescue Remedy for her general irritability. Geraldine calmed down a little and labour was able to proceed smoothly. Twenty minutes later, only two hours after she arrived in the hospital, I was able to deliver her daughter. The time was 12.15 – and I still had time to get to my meeting!

problems during labour and delivery

The majority of women experience a safe, normal labour and birth. However, for a few women situations will develop during the course of the labour which, while not necessarily leading to a complicated birth, may require additional treatment to ensure safe progress. This might include a labour which fails to proceed at the expected pace, delay in the separation and delivery of the placenta (afterbirth), or postpartum haemorrhage.

Slow progress in labour
There are several factors which can contribute to slow progress in labour: the uterus may not work efficiently to dilate the cervix and push the baby downwards; the baby may be in a difficult position from which s/he needs to extricate her/himself before normal progress can be resumed; or the bony pelvis which makes up the birth

canal or passage down which the baby must pass is abnormal in shape or too small. It is important to point out that if the pelvic canal is restricted or has abnormal protruberances inside it which prevent the baby from making the journey outwards, medical care will be needed. It is obviously dangerous to stimulate the uterus artificially to work harder if the reason for the delay in progress is something which cannot be overcome.

Complementary therapies can be used with caution to enhance the uterine contractions on condition that there is no obstruction for the baby through the birth canal. Improving the contractions will indirectly assist in moving the baby into a more favourable position so long as it is already confirmed that the baby is cephalic (head-first). Babies lying sidewards across the uterus are unable to be delivered vaginally and Caesarean section will be necessary. Breech presentation is covered on page 149.

SELF-HELP

- **Aromatherapy** Blends of nutmeg and jasmine may stimulate the uterus to contract better. The oil can be massaged onto your abdomen in a clockwise circular motion. Lavender may also be helpful, but take care with the percentage of the blend as if it is too strong you may feel nauseous. Clary sage can be added to the mix if necessary. For massage, use a maximum of three drops of essential oil in total, diluted in 5ml/ 1 teaspoon of carrier oil; in the bath, use up to six drops of essential oil, diluted as before.
- **Reflexology** Stimulation of the foot zones for the uterus on the midpoint of the inner heel, as well as the specific points for the pituitary gland on the backs of the big toes (see Onset of labour, page 157), triggers the production of more oxytocin hormone to accelerate the uterine action.
- **Shiatsu** The same points as are used to stimulate the onset of labour can be pressed intermittently 20–30 times every 15 minutes (see Onset of labour, page 155).
- **Herbal remedies** Raspberry leaf tea can be sipped throughout labour, even if you have not used it regularly during pregnancy. Squaw vine,

black cohosh or blue cohosh are herbal remedies known to be 'partus preparators' or good for preparing the body for labour. They can be taken in the last few weeks of pregnancy and during labour when progress is slow. It is interesting to note that both black cohosh and blue cohosh are used in homeopathic dilutions for the same purpose.

- **Massage** As with starting labour, stimulation of the nipples through massage will increase the output of oxytocin and encourage more effective contractions.

Homeopathy

The following are just some examples of the ways in which homeopathic remedies can be used to speed up your labour. Take one 30C tablet of the most appropriate remedy every 15 minutes, as required.

- If the contractions have stopped or slowed down because you are frightened, especially if you have a fear of either you or your baby dying; you may have a headache, be restless, have back pain and are very intolerant of internal examinations – aconite.
- If you are putting on a brave face, denying that you are suffering but are in great distress; your body feels cold but your head feels hot, you are restless and sore whatever position you choose, and your contractions are weak and ineffective because the uterus is exhausted – arnica.
- If you are in great distress with a headache, cramps in your legs and hands and a drawing pain from the small of your back to your thighs, making you feel as if your back will break; you are vehemently angry and wildly moaning and thrashing about, wishing to escape, and your face is flushed, hot and with glistening eyes – belladonna.
- If the contractions are weak or stop completely but have a digging and tearing nature when you do experience them; you cannot bear to be touched during a contraction, especially on your hands, and you feel faint, dizzy and exhausted; you feel better if cool fresh air is fanned around you – China.
- If the contractions are spasmodic and ineffectual, mainly in your back and buttocks, and even light touch seems to cause them to stop; you act obstinately and are over-sensitive, restless and feel anxiety in your stomach; your abdomen feels bloated, you are very thirsty and are worn out with a violent headache – kali carb.

- If the contractions are painful but weak, accompanied by shuddering, are spasmodic and shooting upwards from the cervix but you also feel as if you have a weight in your rectum; you are irritable and indifferent, resentful if you are left alone and keep saying you have 'had enough'; you feel as if you want to be covered up to help the pain, have cold extremities but flushes of heat, and feel faint and cold – sepia.

Caesarean section and forceps delivery

Although the majority of mothers achieve a safe, normal, vaginal birth of their babies, problems sometimes arise which necessitate a speedy delivery, either because the baby is in distress or obstructed (stuck) in an abnormal position, or because the mother has become unwell, perhaps haemorrhaging or developing a rapidly rising blood pressure.

A Caesarean section is a major abdominal operation which involves cutting into the uterus to extricate the baby; most women undergo this with the aid of a spinal or epidural anaesthetic, although some will need or request a general anaesthetic. Caesarean sections are either planned or emergency operations.

Elective (planned) Caesareans are performed if either your health or that of your baby could be affected by the exertion of going through normal labour and birth, perhaps due to existing medical conditions or as a result of complications during this or a previous pregnancy, making it safer for the baby to be born in this way. Emergency Caesarean sections are needed if problems occur during labour such as entanglement or prolapse of the baby's umbilical cord, maternal haemorrhage or severe distress of the baby.

Forceps delivery employs the use of metal 'helping hands' which the obstetrician inserts into the vagina and around the head to deliver the baby, and may be needed after the mother has been pushing for a long time in the second stage of labour when the baby's head is low enough in the birth canal to facilitate vaginal delivery. The baby's head may have moved into a position from which it is difficult to manoeuvre further, or s/he may have become tired and distressed from the effort of being born. Occasionally a vacuum extraction is performed, in which a suction cap is applied to the baby's head to pull him/her out without the extra width of forceps inside the vagina, which could cause more trauma.

It is unlikely that, if you are far enough into labour for an operative delivery to be suggested, you will be able to think about appropriate complementary therapies, let alone try using them. It is not feasible at this stage to use complementary strategies to deal with the cause, but they may help to deal with the associated discomforts, perhaps before a planned Caesarean section or following an operative delivery.

SELF-HELP

- **Bach flower remedies** The ubiquitous Rescue Remedy is invaluable just before you go to the operating theatre for a Caesarean section, or at any time during a forceps or vacuum delivery. Four drops neat on your tongue can assist in reducing the anxiety and sense of panic you may feel – and your partner can use it too! It is still possible to use Rescue Remedy despite not being allowed to eat or drink anything as it is literally a few drops, which is no more than a mouthful of saliva. If you are given the choice of a Caesarean section or the opportunity to 'wait and see', you may find it difficult to make a decision and feel the need to seek reassurance from those caring for you. In this case, cerato is useful, or scleranthus. Try rock rose if you feel immense terror and panic, olive for tiredness and mimulus if you are frightened. After the birth you can use walnut to help you adapt to change, olive for the tiredness you will undoubtedly feel, crab apple if you have a sense of uncleanliness, and Star of Bethlehem to overcome the trauma that your body – and mind – has suffered.
- **Breathing exercises** Remember your SOS – Sigh Out Slowly – technique (see page 66) while everything is being prepared for the operation or the forceps/vacuum delivery. If you have practised this at home with your partner during pregnancy, he may also find it usefully distracting to assist in encouraging you with this. You can also repeat these exercises following the birth of your baby, particularly if you have had a general anaesthetic, as they will help to prevent chest infections from developing and facilitate you expanding your lungs fully.
- **Massage** Gentle massage before the delivery can help to take your mind

off the impending operative procedure and relax your muscles, so that your body is enabled to do its work as well as it can. Foot, shoulder or hand massage can be performed by your partner, which can also help him indirectly. In the days following the birth, if you can persuade someone to give you a regular back and shoulder massage your overall well-being will be greatly improved.

- **Aromatherapy** It is not possible to use essential oils in the anaesthetic room before you go into theatre because they are volatile and may interact with the anaesthetic gases (even if you are not having a general anaesthetic, the gases will be in the room). It is unlikely that most hospitals will have considered the value of aromatherapy in the recovery room where you are taken following the Caesarean, although you may be lucky in a few centres. If you are having a planned Caesarean section, you could arrange to receive an aromatherapy massage prior to admission or perhaps immediately before you are moved to the theatre. Citrus oils or ylang ylang, sandalwood or frankincense are relaxing – use a maximum of four drops in total, diluted in 5ml/1 teaspoon of carrier oil. Once you have had the baby, peppermint or spearmint may ease nausea caused by the drugs or anaesthetics – place one or two drops on a cottonwool ball to inhale. Lavender can help with healing and tea tree to reduce the incidence of infections; put three to four drops, diluted in 5ml/1 teaspoon of carrier oil, in the bath once you are allowed to have one.

- **Shiatsu** If the Caesarean section or forceps delivery is being carried out because your baby has become stuck in the birth canal, it is important not to continue with any shiatsu to points which stimulate contractions. This can lead to the uterus trying unsuccessfully to overcome the obstruction and, especially if this is not your first baby, to over-stimulation of the muscles of the uterus, possibly with serious consequences. However, shiatsu techniques for easing sickness are very useful following surgery and acupressure wrist bands or magnets can be used (see Nausea and vomiting, page 71). In the days and weeks following the birth you may appreciate an energizing shiatsu treatment to help you overcome the after-effects of the surgery.

- **Reflexology** Similarly, reflexology manipulations which encourage uterine contractions should be omitted but simple holding of the heels, very firmly, can ease some of the pain if you are continuing to contract while waiting for the forceps or Caesarean delivery. This works on the areas of the feet related to the uterus and pelvic region and can also be relaxing at a time when you will be feeling anxious. One of the problems following abdominal surgery is an inability to have the bowels open due to the intestines temporarily going into spasm – and reflexology is wonderful for relieving this. Clockwise massage of the arches of the feet will suffice, and will enable you to commence eating again as soon as possible.

Homeopathy

The two most useful remedies are arnica for shock, trauma and bruising, and hypericum to aid healing. (For homeopathic remedies you can use to combat the effects of drugs used, see page 117.)

- If the surgery is planned, take one 30C tablet of each remedy the night before, and one of each on the morning of the delivery.
- For the first 24 hours following surgery, take one tablet of each remedy every hour (while awake).
- For the second 24 hours, take one tablet of each remedy every 2 hours.
- For the third 24 hours, take one tablet of each remedy every 3 hours.
- Stop after the third day.

OTHER THERAPIES WHICH MAY HELP

For these therapies, refer to a qualified practitioner.

Cranial osteopathy may be appropriate. Some osteopaths believe that babies born by forceps delivery are more likely to suck their thumbs, because the forceps blades place an abnormal pressure around the baby's head during the birth. This then leads to tensions in the brain which contribute to the headaches that babies delivered by forceps are thought to suffer. In an attempt to relieve this internal pressure, the baby spontaneously sucks his/her thumb, directing the force of the thumb upwards and backwards to the upper palate in the mouth. Treatment to reduce this pressure at an early stage following forceps delivery may avoid the long-term effects of thumb sucking such as misaligned teeth.

Osteopathy or **chiropractic** can be relaxing for you and is especially useful if you have had a forceps delivery in which your legs would have been put up in lithotomy stirrups. These can cause displacement of your hips and spine, and treatment from a qualified practitioner can assist in aligning your joints and bones once again.

Acupuncture has been used instead of general anaesthetic for Caesarean sections, although mostly in China where acupuncture is a normal complement to conventional care and it is highly unlikely that you would be able to arrange this elsewhere. However, you may be able to have a qualified acupuncturist in attendance to provide pain relief, ease nausea and vomiting, and help you cope with anxiety. Following delivery, rebalancing of your energies may help to avoid the minor complications which can occur after operations including nausea and vomiting, abdominal distension and pain.

Pre-term labour

A pre-term or premature labour is one which occurs before the thirty-seventh week of pregnancy, before the baby is grown and mature enough to be fully capable of existing outside the uterine environment without medical help. It may be that labour begins spontaneously due to trauma, such as an accident, over-stretching of the uterus caused by excessive fluid or more than one baby, or as a result of high temperature and infection such as a kidney infection. Sometimes there is an early spontaneous rupture of the bag of membranes surrounding the baby, which often leads to contractions. Alternatively, labour may be started early artificially because medical staff believe the condition of the mother or baby will be better once the baby is out of the uterus – this may be in situations where the mother has suffered excessive bleeding, very high blood pressure or the baby is simply not thriving inside the uterus.

Pre-term labour always requires medical supervision. Spontaneous onset of pre-term labour may require the use of special drugs to attempt to stop the contractions and delay the birth of the immature baby. Where labour has been started prematurely because of medical complications, treatment focuses on monitoring the progress and condition of the baby and preparing for his/her birth, when neonatal intensive care may be needed.

This section does not deal with situations where labour has been induced deliberately, although you could refer to other relevant sections for using complementary therapies for relaxation, pain and aftercare. Any complementary treatment provided for mothers whose labours have started spontaneously must be given in consultation with medical and midwifery staff to avoid additional complications, which may arise as a result of interactions between natural remedies and conventional drugs. However, you may find some of these suggestions helpful if you have a history of pre-term labour in a previous pregnancy.

SELF-HELP

- **Bach flower remedies** You will naturally be extremely anxious and can use Rescue Remedy for general relief of anxiety. If you have had an accident or fall which has triggered pre-term labour you can take Star of Bethlehem and rock rose, two drops of each three times daily, to ease your emotional state. If you are excessively concerned for the welfare of your baby, try red chestnut. Walnut, for helping you to deal with the impending change to your life, is also useful. If you are very frightened, try mimulus or aspen.

- **Aromatherapy** It is my opinion that you should refrain from using essential oils while you are contracting in pre-term labour, even if it seems that your labour will not stop but will proceed to delivery. Many of the oils useful for relieving pain in labour will also stimulate contractions; those which are too strong can squeeze a premature baby excessively and cause more distress than is already present. If contractions stop and pregnancy continues you will also need to be careful in using essential oils, as your uterus will now be more susceptible to any factors which may trigger labour. Very low dilutions of oils (no more than two drops in 5ml/1 teaspoon of carrier oil) can be used in the bath to reduce blood pressure – rather than lavender, I would suggest rosewood or camomile – but *not* if your membranes have ruptured. If this is a pregnancy subsequent to a previous pre-term labour, you could use low doses (two or three drops in 5ml/1 teaspoon of carrier oil) of citrus oils, ylang ylang and camomile for relaxation.

- **Nutritional therapy** There are many reasons why some women go into labour prematurely, but it is certainly known that dietary factors can play a part in preventing the problem from recurring. Smoking and alcohol intake are known to cause pre-term labour and you should make every effort to stop or cut down. Maintaining adequate levels of vitamins and minerals, particularly zinc, magnesium, calcium and essential fatty acids, may be beneficial in preventing the problem. If necessary, supplements of calcium gluconate (1–2g daily) and magnesium (500–700mg daily) can be taken, as well as 2–3g of evening primrose oil each day, although you should avoid the latter if you are epileptic.
- **Relaxation techniques, Tai Chi** and **yoga** If you have a history of pre-term labour in a previous pregnancy you should make every effort to reduce stress, which is known to trigger early contractions. Try gentle swimming, Tai Chi, yoga and breathing exercises – and get plenty of rest, especially around the time when labour started in the previous pregnancy.

Homeopathy

Unless otherwise stated, take one 30C tablet of the most appropriate remedy every hour while contractions continue.

- If early contractions have been brought on by an accident or traumatic incident; you may feel bruised and sore in any position and constantly want to change it; you want to be left alone and do not like being examined – arnica. Take one 30C tablet three times daily.
- If labour begins at about 28–32 weeks of pregnancy; you feel irritable, easily angered but may also be weepy; you experience shuddering during contractions and want to be covered; you are likely to have had several babies or two close together – sepia.
- If excessive nausea and vomiting has led to pre-term labour; you feel worse lying down and feel sharp, cutting pains around your umbilicus – ipecacuanha.
- If there are no other indications for another remedy; you may have a history of headaches or arthritic-type problems; you experience nervous chills and shivering in the first stage of labour – cimicifuga.
- If your emotions are prominent, you are emotionally restless, have grave fears

and concerns for your baby and need a lot of reassurance and support; you burst into tears easily; your baby's movements feel violent and painful and you are intolerant of being in a warm room – pulsatilla.

OTHER THERAPIES WHICH MAY HELP

For these therapies, refer to a qualified practitioner.

Shiatsu, massage and **reflexology** can all be extremely relaxing; you could try some techniques yourself or visit a qualified therapist. However, it is important not to stimulate the points which can trigger labour (see Onset of labour, page 153).

Retained placenta and haemorrhage following delivery

The third stage of labour involves the separation of the placenta from the lining of the uterus, followed by its expulsion. The muscle layer of the uterus should then contract in order to prevent haemorrhage. Occasionally the placenta is slow to separate, perhaps because the uterus is tired after either a very long labour or one which was so quick that the force of contractions has exhausted the muscles. If nature is left to take its course the placenta will separate and be expelled, usually in about 20–30 minutes, but the process can take as long as two hours. However, if only a partial separation occurs, so that some of the placenta remains attached to the lining of the uterus, more serious bleeding can occur. This is called primary postpartum haemorrhage if it happens immediately after the baby's birth or during the first 24 hours. If the placenta fails to separate at all, it will need to be removed in a manual operation while you are given a general anaesthetic, because the risks of later bleeding are too great.

Certain complementary strategies can be employed to encourage the uterus to contract fully, so that the whole placenta is squeezed off the lining wall and can then be pushed or pulled out. Complete emptying of your uterus cannot be guaranteed but every effort is made to ensure that no clots are left behind, in an attempt to avoid the need for the manual removal. You may also be asked to try to pass urine, as a full bladder can prevent the uterus from clamping down sufficiently.

- **Massage** your two nipples between finger and thumb to produce oxytocin to trigger a more effective contraction, or better still, put your baby to the breast to suckle.

  Gentle abdominal massage of the top of your uterus may be carried out by your midwife or doctor – this encourages the muscles of the uterus to contract, in which case the top of the uterus becomes rock hard and the placenta is forced off the lining wall.

- **Reflexology** Ask your partner or birth companion to massage the middle of your inner heels on both feet – this is where the reflex zone for the uterus is situated. Also try intermittent pressure on the backs of the big toes, which are the zones for the pituitary gland – you will know if you are on the right spot as it will be very sharply painful. (For both points, see fig. 4, page 209.)

- **Aromatherapy** Quickly put two drops of jasmine, nutmeg or basil essential oil onto a cottonwool ball and inhale the vapours, as this can trigger contractions. Alternatively, you could ask someone to massage the oil (diluted in 5ml/1 teaspoon of carrier oil) into your abdomen or feet.

- **Shiatsu** Ask your partner to press the Bl67 point on your little toe or the Li4 point in the webbing of your thumb and forefinger; press intermittently about 20–30 times (see Onset of labour, page 155).

- **Herbal remedies** If you already have raspberry leaf tea available, drink whatever remains as this may initiate contraction of your uterus.

Homeopathy

Take one 30C or 6C tablet of the most appropriate remedy every five minutes, as required.

- If there are no contractions, the placenta is partially separated and there is profuse bleeding of dark red blood; you feel weak, exhausted and trembling – caulophyllum.

- If your uterus fails to contract, blood loss is dark but without clots and you feel sharp, shooting pains in the area of your cervix; you also feel faint, have flushes of heat but your hands and feet are cold and may feel better if you draw up your legs – sepia.

- If you have no contractions, the placenta remains high up in your uterus and your abdomen is painful if touched; there is continued pain but bleeding is intermittent and you are unable to pass urine when requested to try; you feel restless and tearful, need air and have a sensation of heat and soreness just below your ribs, especially on the right side – pulsatilla. This remedy can also be used if there is no clear indication for another remedy.

OTHER THERAPIES WHICH MAY HELP

For these therapies, refer to a qualified practitioner.

Osteopathy or **chiropractic** techniques can be helpful if a practitioner is in attendance, to facilitate separation and expulsion of the placenta.

Acupuncture needles can be inserted into the main points used to trigger labour to encourage contraction of the uterus and separation of the placenta. If haemorrhage continues, acupuncture can also assist in controlling it.

6

mother and baby

Whether or not this is your first time, becoming a new mother is an exciting, fascinating, wonderful time for most women, but it is certainly not all 'plain sailing' for many. You will be beset by numerous worries and concerns at a time when you are recovering physically from the pregnancy and delivery, establishing your routine and feeding method for your baby, as well as coming to terms with the awesome responsibility of parenthood.

In these first few days and weeks you will also experience a range of other physical and emotional discomforts as your body returns to the non-pregnant state, most of which are caused by fluctuating hormone levels (again). This chapter provides a few suggestions for dealing with the common complaints that may affect you and some of the minor conditions your baby may develop. Some of the problems you suffer may already have been troublesome during pregnancy, for example constipation, and you should refer to the relevant section for advice regarding complementary therapies which may be appropriate for dealing with these.

breast changes

Once the baby and the placenta have been delivered, the pregnancy hormone levels in your body fall dramatically and other hormones that are responsible for lactation are released from the pituitary gland in the brain to initiate milk production. Although the nutritious colostrum (pre-milk) is present, your main milk supply will normally come into your breasts by about the third day after the birth, irrespective of whether you are breastfeeding or not. Unfortunately, this happens at a time when your hormone levels are also having an impact on your moods and you are prone to postnatal 'blues' (see page 198), your perineum may be throbbing, especially if you have had stitches (see Care of your perineum, page 181), and your baby recovers from the ordeal of being born and starts to make his/her presence felt – loudly!

When to seek further advice
This section is not specifically about assisting you with breastfeeding your baby, as you will be given help by the midwives and maternity nurses. Fixing your baby onto the nipple properly is the best means of preventing sore nipples, but you may still experience some soreness in the early days. When the milk first comes into your breasts you may suffer engorgement until the amount is balanced out by the baby's sucking: eventually supply will equal demand. Occasionally mastitis develops, in which the breast becomes inflamed, hot and sore to touch; if left untreated this can go on to become a breast abscess, so it is important to seek medical help as well as continuing to use the relevant complementary therapies.

SELF-HELP

- **Nutritional therapy** Garlic has been found to increase the time for which a baby sucks at the breast, which helps to empty the breast fully and prevent mastitis. Babies also appear to suck more efficiently when the milk is flavoured with garlic! Eating plenty of fresh, even raw, garlic will assist in this process and help prevent infections. Oats, in the form of porridge, lift the spirits and encourage a good milk supply. It is imperative to drink plenty of fluids throughout the day – you will probably feel very thirsty – and to eat a diet rich in proteins, vitamins and minerals. 'Eating for two' is certainly true during breastfeeding, though not a good idea in pregnancy.

- **Herbal remedies** Make a tea from fennel seeds and sip it throughout the day to stimulate your milk supply. Nettle tea may also help. If you develop sore nipples, use camomile teabags which have been steeped in boiling water, cooled and squeezed out. Apply one teabag to each nipple and put your bra on over the top. Camomile contains chemicals which are pain-relieving and anti-inflammatory. You may be able to obtain a commercial cream containing camomile which can be rubbed onto your nipples for the same purpose, but you will need to wash this off gently before your baby goes to the breast to avoid him/her ingesting it. Alternatively, geranium (*Pelargonium*) leaves placed inside the bra against your nipples – underside nearest the skin – will ease the soreness. If you develop engorgement, try the leaves of a dark green cabbage inside your bra. This draws heat from your breasts and relieves the excess swelling. Change the cabbage leaves whenever they become wet and limp. You could also try a cold poultice of grated raw potato or carrot, or a hot poultice of parsley. Tie together a bunch of parsley, simmer in water for ten minutes, then cool to a comfortable temperature before applying to your breasts.

- **Massage** Nipple massage before delivery can help you to become accustomed to handling your breasts for feeding your baby; it can also encourage flat nipples to protrude outwards to facilitate the baby latching on properly. Five minutes daily on each nipple separately for the last three to four weeks of pregnancy will be sufficient. If your breasts become engorged, try massaging gently from your armpit down towards the nipple, using both hands. This encourages the flow of milk and prevents stasis in the milk ducts, which can lead to mastitis.

- **Aromatherapy** Essential oils should not be applied to your breasts if you are breastfeeding unless you wipe them off before the baby goes to suck. There is some evidence that geranium oil helps in cases of engorgement but the dose should be kept to a minimum – about two drops in 5ml/1 teaspoon of carrier oil, which is then massaged into the breasts. Jasmine has been found in two research trials to be capable of suppressing lactation if you are not intending to breastfeed, although you may find it more convenient to drink jasmine tea. Note that this research contradicts much of what is written in general interest aromatherapy books, which often surmise that jasmine will actually stimulate milk production.

- **Reflexology** This therapy can be performed on the hands as well as on the feet, and this is a simple technique that you could do for yourself: massage the tops of your hands nearest the fingers and across the bony knuckles, which are the hand reflexology zones for the breasts.

- **Bach flower remedies** Establishing breastfeeding for the first time can be time consuming, frustrating, tiring and painful, but is well worth the effort – if you survive the first week, you should be able to continue breastfeeding for as long as you wish. Use Rescue Remedy when you feel exasperated and frustrated, larch if you fear failure with your breastfeeding, or oak if you are completely overwhelmed by exhaustion despite a real desire to succeed. If you have a setback in your routine of feeding, or if a complication arises when you were doing well, try gentian, and if you feel totally discouraged and full of despair, use gorse. If you feel impatient with yourself or your baby, use impatiens.

- **Relaxation techniques** It is important to remain as calm and relaxed as possible when you are feeding your baby, whether on the breast or by bottle. Use your SOS – Sigh Out Slowly – breathing (see page 66), especially if it is the middle of the night and you feel you do not have the patience to continue.

- **Positioning** This is vital to the success of feeding your baby and applies whether you are breast- or bottlefeeding. Make sure you are well supported with adequate cushions so that you can lift your baby to your breast, rather than stooping down to put your breast to the baby's mouth. This will prevent you from developing a pain in your neck or between your shoulder blades. Attend to your stitches if you have any – sitting uncomfortably on a sore perineum is one of the most common reasons for discontinuing breastfeeding (see Care of your perineum, page 181).

Homeopathy for breastfeeding difficulties

The following are just a few examples of how homeopathy can be used to relieve breastfeeding problems; more specific help can be obtained from a qualified practitioner. Take one 30C tablet of the most appropriate remedy three times daily for three days.

- If you have inadequate lactation, your breasts are lumpy and sensitive when touched, and your nipples are cracked, burning and itching; the problem is worst after midnight and you do not like being on your own – arsenicum.
- If there is either inadequate or excessive lactation, acute swelling around your nipples with a burning pain which is worse in the right breast; you may have mastitis, with your breasts being inflamed, engorged, tender, hot and throbbing; they may appear bright red and shiny and have red streaks from the centre to the edges – belladonna.
- If your breasts are pale, despite being hot, engorged and inflamed; they feel stony, hard and heavy as lead, and tender, and you experience pain on the slightest movement, worse in the left breast; you may have a temperature, feel sick and thirsty, and often develop a headache after feeding your baby; you may have either insufficient or too much milk – bryonia.
- If you are not feeding your baby but have developed mastitis while the milk supply attempts to dry up, or if you have had a breast infection and now have insufficient milk; your nipples may be cracked and burning and your breasts feel stretched and intensely sore; the pain extends to your chest, neck and back, and you feel weepy, particularly while feeding, and you have a pain in your uterus at this time – pulsatilla.
- If your milk supply is poor or excessive; your nipples are cracked and bleeding and may be inverted, and you feel a cutting pain inside them; your breasts are inflamed, deep red with pale rose-coloured edges and you experience pain during feeding, worse in the left breast, which extends to your shoulder; you get incredibly hot at night, are constipated, have back pain and a headache after feeding – silica.

OTHER THERAPIES WHICH MAY HELP

For these therapies, refer to a qualified practitioner.

Acupuncture and **shiatsu** both work on rebalancing your energies, which have been drained during the birth. An acupuncturist will attempt to induce deep relaxation to help you overcome any tensions which may be inhibiting your milk supply. It has also been shown in research trials that acupuncture encourages the production of the body's own relaxing chemicals as well as other hormones, including those responsible for milk production. A shiatsu practitioner would work the length of the Stomach, Spleen and Kidney meridians in order to build up the most appropriate energy levels.

Osteopathy or **chiropractic** can help postnatally to release tensions in the spine which may be affecting the output of lactation hormones from the pituitary gland in the brain.

Reflexology, stimulating the foot zones related to the breasts, as well as those for the pituitary gland from which the lactation hormones are produced, will facilitate lactation and can be used if there is insufficient milk supply. Reflexology is also useful for helping relieve the discomfort of engorgement by encouraging the flow of milk.

care of your perineum

You may be fortunate enough to have had a normal vaginal delivery without any trauma to your vagina, vulva or perineum, although it is more probable that, even if you do not need stitches, you will have some grazing, bruising and soreness in the area. If you have a normal vaginal delivery you may suffer a small tear of your perineum, but if you have a forceps or vacuum delivery you will almost certainly have undergone an episiotomy (a cut to enlarge the birth opening).

Your vagina and vulva will feel sore for some time and may feel worse when you pass urine as it runs over the stitch line, and your buttocks may be bruised, especially if you have had a forceps delivery. Having your bowels open or having sex for the first time after delivery can also be fraught with fears about pain and discomfort (see 'Private and personal', page 187). It is a good idea to have attempted full intercourse by the time of your six-week check after the birth, so that any major complications as a result of poor healing can be dealt with promptly. Complementary therapies can be used to ease some of the discomfort and aid healing.

When to seek further advice

If you experience severe pain either inside the vagina or on the outer surface of the vulva you may have an infection developing or, rarely, a haematoma, which is a collection of blood beneath the surface of the skin rather like a very large bruise. In this case, you will need to consult your doctor for the haematoma to be drained. If you become aware of any stitches remaining after about a month you should inform your doctor when you have your six-week postnatal check.

SELF-HELP

- **Massage** Perineal massage with almond or avocado oil in the antenatal period will help to facilitate stretching of the perineum in labour and avoid too much damage (see Well-being during pregnancy, page 147). Massage can also be used to relax you before penetration during intercourse, whether this is locally around your vagina and vulva or more generally.
- **Aromatherapy** Essential oils can be added to the bath or bidet as an aid to relieving pain and discomfort and to prevent infection. A trial in one maternity unit investigated the use of lavender oil, as it has long been advocated as an aid to wound healing. This was not borne out by the research, which found that the speed of healing was no quicker in mothers who used the lavender than in those who did not. However, it was discovered that the lavender acted as a reasonable pain-reliever and helped to relax the mothers. Tea tree can be combined with the lavender if there are signs of infection. Camomile, thyme or geranium oils may also be beneficial. Use a maximum of four drops of your chosen oil(s), diluted in 5ml/1 teaspoon of carrier oil.
- **Bach flower remedies** Crab apple is valuable if you feel generally unclean, while Rescue Remedy cream can be applied to sore buttocks, although not directly over an open wound. If the tenderness in the vulval

area makes you feel irritable, try impatiens. Your midwife will need to examine your perineum from time to time to ensure that it is healing properly; if you feel embarrassed and inhibited, water violet is useful.

- **Hydrotherapy** Soothing the perineal wound area with water is one of the simplest remedies. Use the bidet or sit in a shallow bath of warm or cool water, according to your preference. You could use a vulval wash by pouring warm water down over the area from a jug: this is good if you are confined to bed for any reason. However, jacuzzis should not be used because the chemicals may be harmful and the water from the jets could forcibly enter your vagina and uterus, potentially causing a condition called air embolus. This acts rather like a clot which blocks a blood vessel when a stroke or heart attack occurs, and can be very serious.

- **Nutritional therapy** Wound healing will be helped by a nourishing diet including foods which contain zinc and iron, plus vitamins B and C. Eat plenty of fruit and vegetables and drink large quantities of fluid. (See also Well-being in pregnancy, page 146.)

- **Herbal remedies** If your perineum is swollen or bruised, you can make a warm decoction of oak and comfrey barks to which is added an infusion of marigold and lavender flowers. If there is damage to the deeper muscle layers or there is a risk of infection, you should add 15ml/1 dessertspoon each of slippery elm and golden seal powders. This whole cocktail is then diluted in a bowl of warm water large enough for you to sit in and soak the affected area for 20–30 minutes; repeat the process daily until relief is obtained. A witch hazel compress is also quite effective.

- **Relaxation techniques** Although these will not directly ease pain or aid healing, breathing exercises can be helpful prior to opening your bowels, or before penetration the first time you have sex following the birth.

Homeopathy

Take one 30C tablet of the most appropriate remedy three times daily for three days.

- Arnica is the most universal remedy for episiotomy, tears and other trauma. The dosage given above will be sufficient for trauma following a normal delivery. An arnica cream is also available; it should not be applied to the stitch line or an open wound, but can be rubbed gently into bruised areas. If you have had a forceps delivery or vacuum extraction, follow the regime on page 169.

- Calendula tablets can be taken after episiotomy, when the skin is broken and the pain is more than the wound size would seem to warrant. As with arnica, a cream is available which can be applied to an open wound, or the tincture can be added to a glass of water and applied to the wound.
- If the pain makes it almost impossible to walk and is worse when the weather changes or if you drink coffee but better if you have cold drinks; you may feel emotionally sad and frightened – causticum.
- After episiotomy and following unpleasant examinations or catheterization, if you experience a feeling of humiliation, anger and indignation; you feel worse if you are touched or when you have exerted yourself – staphysagria.

OTHER THERAPIES WHICH MAY HELP
For these therapies, refer to a qualified practitioner.
Reflexology, using careful and precise suppression of the specific foot zones related to the vagina and perineum, can help to relieve pain.
Acupuncture for overall relaxation may afford some relief, and specific points can be worked to ease pain.

vaginal blood loss and after-pains

Following the birth of your baby you will experience some vaginal blood loss, like a very heavy period; initially this is bright red, then progresses to a brownish loss and finally to a yellowish discharge, which usually lasts for about ten days but may persist for some weeks. This loss is the remaining tissues from the placenta as well as the lining of the uterus, which must be shed before your menstrual cycle recommences.

When you are examined each day following your baby's birth, the midwife needs to ensure not only that your loss is normal but also that your uterus is shrinking back down to its non-pregnant size, shape and position. This process is called involution and the midwife will assess your progress by feeling the top of your uterus via your abdomen. When the top of the uterus can no longer be felt above the pubic bone, the process of involution is almost complete. Occasionally this process is slow (sub-involution), perhaps because there are retained clots and bits of placenta inside, or if your uterus was excessively stretched – perhaps if you had a big baby, or twins, or excess fluid.

You may experience 'after-pains' in your uterus, especially while you are breastfeeding, as the hormones which produce milk also make your uterus contract. These pains may be minor if this is your first baby, but can be quite uncomfortable if you have had several babies or your uterus has been stretched by a large baby, excess fluid or more than one baby.

When to seek further advice

If your blood loss is red and then stops suddenly you should notify your midwife as, surprisingly, this may signify an imminent haemorrhage. If the discharge contains large clots of blood you should also inform your midwife, because this too could indicate that a small part of placenta has been left behind in the uterus. Save any clots passed for the midwife to examine. If the loss begins to smell offensive at any time this could indicate infection as well as retained products, and you may require antibiotics. If the after-pains are very severe your body may be attempting to rid itself of extra-large clots or pieces of the placenta, so it is advisable to inform your midwife.

SELF-HELP

- **Aromatherapy** As with care of your perineum (see page 182), aromatherapy can be used to help keep the area clean and free from infection; lavender, camomile and tea tree are good for this. If sub-involution occurs you can use clary sage or jasmine in your bath, as these will help the uterus to contract down to expel any clots or tissues left behind. However, you must use a low dose of essential oil (no more than two drops diluted in 5ml/1 teaspoon of carrier oil) to prevent triggering a major haemorrhage. Geranium is best avoided if you have had any serious blood loss, as it may possibly interfere with clotting mechanisms. Two drops of lavender in 5ml/1 teaspoon of carrier oil, massaged carefully into your abdomen, can help to relieve after-pains.

- **Bach flower remedies** You may wish to use four drops of crab apple in your bathwater to reduce the feeling of uncleanliness, or take two drops, three times daily, until you feel better. If you suffer a haemorrhage, when you may become anaemic and will feel very tired, use olive, and if you have a haemorrhage or sub-involution, in particular when you were previously doing well and now feel you have suffered a setback, you could try gentian.
- **Reflexology** As with retained placenta (see page 174), intermittent pressure applied to the two points on the backs of the big toes that represent the pituitary gland will cause more oxytocin hormone to be produced, which will facilitate expulsion of any retained products. The part of the inner heel related to the uterus can also be stimulated. (For both points, see fig. 4, page 209.)
- **Herbal remedies** If you have any raspberry leaf tea or tablets left from your pregnancy you can finish this up, drinking one cup three times daily, simply as a preventative measure. If heavy bleeding occurs or there is sub-involution, you can use lady's mantle, freshly picked shepherd's purse or nettles, in teas or tinctures.

Homeopathy

Take one 30C tablet of the most appropriate remedy three times daily for three days.

- If you have pains shooting down into your hips, buttocks and legs with stitch-like contractions, backache and heavy perspiring; you feel touchy, angry and irritable – kali carb.
- If you have very little blood loss, your uterus remains high (sub-involution) and after-pains are changeable in nature; emotionally you are also changeable, you are tired, weepy and restless and have a bad taste in your mouth but are not thirsty; you feel better when out in the fresh air and worse if in a stuffy room – pulsatilla.
- If your blood loss suddenly becomes dark brown and offensive-smelling; you have prolonged but irregular bearing-down contractions which are worse while

you are breastfeeding; you look pale and feel cold but want to be uncovered and feel very anxious (this situation is most likely if you have had four or more babies) – secale.

■ If your blood flow increases with every contraction and is hot and offensive, but generally scanty; you feel worse for any jarring movements and around 3pm, but better if you are lying down; you are excitable and confused, hot and flushed – belladonna.

OTHER THERAPIES WHICH MAY HELP

For these therapies, refer to a qualified practitioner.

Acupuncture or **shiatsu**, focusing on the same points that are used to stimulate labour contractions, can assist in expelling clots and retained products, which in turn facilitates the natural process of involution.

Osteopathy or **chiropractic** may possibly be useful if after-pains persist, by releasing tensions contributing to poor emptying of your uterus.

'private and personal'

It may seem, once you are pregnant, in labour or newly delivered, that there is no privacy left to you, for every private and personal aspect of your life appears to be under scrutiny, even your sex life and going to the toilet. As you become occupied with caring for your new baby, you will also feel that you have no time to attend to these intimate aspects. However, any, or all, of these matters, if left unattended, can cause you at best discomfort, and in the worst cases serious problems. It is therefore important to ensure that you have sufficient time and privacy to empty your bladder fully and regularly, to evacuate your bowels properly to avoid constipation, and to share the intimacies with your partner which were a part of your relationship before your baby was born.

Immediately after the birth you will find that you are constantly passing urine, in large quantities. This is because all the extra tissues, muscles, blood vessels and so on which were grown during pregnancy to provide food and oxygen for your baby need to be excreted from your body. These tissues are dissolved into fluid in the blood vessels and eventually reach the kidneys, to be passed out as urine. Initially, however, there is too much fluid for the kidneys to deal with at one time and you may suffer increased swelling in your ankles and feet until the excess fluid has been lost. There is an increased tendency towards urinary infection and hygiene is important, especially while you are still losing blood. Occasionally, problems with passing urine immediately after delivery, as a result of bruising of the bladder and ureters, can lead to retention of urine, which can be very uncomfortable and precipitate infection. Incontinence of urine (and occasionally faeces) can be a long-term problem for some women due to over-stretching of and damage to the pelvic floor muscles.

It is often very uncomfortable having your bowels open for the first time after your baby's birth, especially if you have stitches or haemorrhoids or have been constipated at the end of pregnancy. Fear of discomfort can make it an even more painful experience. A change in your diet, especially if you are in hospital for several days, may affect your bowels and cause constipation. In addition, the nerves in the anus and the area of your perineum will have suffered some trauma during delivery, which can reduce the sensation of needing to have your bowels open and add to any difficulties you may have.

Is there sex after childbirth?! In the months to come you may ask yourself this frequently, as the demands of breastfeeding and caring for your baby, and the overwhelming sense of tiredness you will feel, take over your entire being.

The suggestions given here for using complementary therapies may help to ease these situations (see also Constipation, page 75, and Problems with sex, page 109).

SELF-HELP

- **Massage** Clockwise abdominal massage may stimulate intestinal movement to encourage a bowel movement. If loss of sensation means that you are unable to pass out a motion which is in the rectum, you can carefully insert a clean thumb into your vagina and massage the back wall which rests against the rectum, to move the stool further down towards the anal opening. Gentle massage above your pubic bone may help to encourage your flow of urine. Sensual body massage is a pleasant way of enjoying intimacy prior to intercourse. Perineal and clitoral massage can encourage production of natural lubricants from within the vagina, for dryness is often an added problem after childbirth. (The use of commercial lubricants is not recommended unless they are specifically indicated as suitable for *vaginal* dryness.)

- **Aromatherapy** Citrus oils such as tangerine, mandarin, sweet orange, neroli, bergamot, lime, grapefruit and lemon, in any combination, added to the bath or used in a massage blend as above, can work on the digestive tract to prevent constipation. Sandalwood and camomile oils seem to have an affinity with the urinary tract and can be used in a compress pressed against the area just above the pubic bone, or on the back of the hips over the kidneys if there is any suspicion of infection, or added to 0.5 litre of warm water and used as a vulval wash to ease the irritation of urine passing over the stitch line. Sandalwood is also thought to be an aphrodisiac, as are ylang ylang and rose oils, and all help to increase the sense of relaxation which in itself can facilitate intimacy. For all these uses, add a maximum of four drops of essential oil to 5ml/1 teaspoon of carrier oil.

- **Bach flower remedies** If you are fearful of having your bowels open, or of that first postnatal sexual contact, use two drops of mimulus. If you are weary and unable to find the energy for sex, olive or hornbeam may be useful, or if you normally keep going but are currently overwhelmed with exhaustion, use oak. If you are over-concerned about your baby and cannot find time for yourself, take red chestnut and rock water. If the effort of having your bowels open leaves you sweating and worn out, take four drops of Rescue Remedy, before sitting on the toilet as well as afterwards.

- **Herbal remedies** Camomile tea is one of the most effective of the antiseptic herbal remedies which work on the urinary system. Drink several cups daily, as this will assist in the prevention of urinary infection and also relax you. (See also the suggestions for herbal remedies for Constipation, page 76, and Urinary symptoms, page 107.)

- **Nutritional therapy** Obviously a good diet is vital to the overall healing process of recovering from the birth, and general suggestions for healthy eating can be found on page 146. In order to prevent both constipation and urinary infection, you should attempt to drink at least 3–4 litres of water each day. You may like to consider using food as a means of relaxing you prior to attempting sex for the first time. Make time for yourselves so that it is an 'occasion', ask someone else to look after your baby for a while, perhaps overnight, and prepare a delicious meal of all the delicacies you like to eat. Better still, choose 'nibbles' and feed each other in bed!

- **Relaxation techniques** Deep breathing exercises will help you open your bowels when there is no sensation. In this, as in sex, it is vital to allocate sufficient time to complete the process – incomplete emptying of your bowels can lead to long-term constipation. Privacy is also important: you may not feel mentally and physically comfortable enough while you are still in a hospital ward to spend the requisite amount of time on the toilet. Breathe deeply and relax your pelvic floor muscles to open the anus, then bear down gently, but do not strain. Relaxation exercises can also help at the point of penetration during sex if you are particularly tense, as this will help to open up your vagina. Pelvic floor exercises (see page 196) are essential to prevent long-term problems such as urinary or faecal incontinence, sexual difficulties or prolapse of your uterus.

- **Positioning** If opening your bowels is difficult, try standing over the toilet with one foot on a chair or the bath, as this can relax and open up your pelvic floor area. Leaning forwards may also help. When passing urine, it may feel less sensitive to squat forwards to direct the flow straight down into the toilet, rather than letting the urine run down over your perineum and across the stitches. When trying sex for the first few times after the birth, adapt your positions to take pressure off wherever you feel most discomfort. This may be the front of your vagina if you have a lot of grazes, or around your perineum and anus if you have several stitches. If you have had a Caesarean section, you may need to be on top to avoid pressure on your wound; very deep intercourse may also be out of the question initially. Anal sex is not recommended at this stage because of the increased risk of transferring infection from the anus to the vagina.

Homeopathy for postnatal urinary problems

Take one 30C tablet of the most appropriate remedy three times daily for three days.

- If you have either retention or incontinence, especially after a prolonged labour or difficult birth such as a forceps delivery; passing urine is painful and sore and causes pressure in your bladder, and you may involuntarily pass some urine when asleep or running or coughing; you dislike being touched and deny that you are suffering – arnica.
- If you are unable to pass urine following delivery, have an ineffectual urge and a constant bearing-down pressure; you feel a severe back pain before you pass urine but this is eased once you are able to go, although the flow of urine is not very strong; you cry before starting to pass urine – lycopodium.
- If you are unable to pass urine or find yourself passing small amounts frequently but only a little at a time and very slowly; the urine is rather acrid-smelling, pale and watery and feels as if it is burning; you feel very pessimistic but better if you drink cold fluids – causticum.
- If you cannot pass urine but have no desire to do so either; there is burning pain and when you do pass any urine this also feels as if it is burning; the urine may contain blood or pus and may be dark yellow, brownish or greenish in colour; you feel anxious, restless and fearful; the problem is worse when coughing or after exertion but better if you are hot – arsenicum.
- If you find it difficult to pass urine or have a constant dribbling, and you have a shooting pain in the kidney area; your urine is copious, pale and watery or may be turbid, yellowish-red and you may pass faeces at the same time; the problem is worse at night – belladonna.

OTHER THERAPIES WHICH MAY HELP

For these therapies, refer to a qualified practitioner.

Acupuncture can relieve constipation, assist the passage of urine if you are unable to empty your bladder, ease the pain of haemorrhoids and generally relax you. The UB57 point on the back of the calf (see fig. 4, page 209) lies on the bladder meridian which passes around the anus and is a particularly effective point for dealing with haemorrhoids. Inserting needles into points on the lower legs as well as above the symphysis pubis (pubic bones) can help in treating retention of urine.

Reflexology using specific techniques can treat retention of urine, constipation and haemorrhoids. It will also increase the production of encephalins and endorphins, the body's natural antidepressants from the brain, which will help to relax you in preparation for intercourse again.

Osteopathy or **chiropractic**, using manipulation of the spine and muscles, may succeed in releasing tensions contributing to urinary symptoms, especially around the ureters leading from the kidneys to the bladder.

Hypnotherapy can be useful if, in the longer term, sexual activity is affected by your inability to relax sufficiently to facilitate penetration, as it may help you to overcome the subconscious fears and inhibitions affecting your sex life.

general aches and discomforts

Establishing breastfeeding and coping with your blood loss, bowels, waterworks and return to sexual activity are all natural consequences of having been pregnant as your body returns to the non-pregnant state. However, labour itself can be a factor in some of the discomforts you may experience, such as when you have received drugs for pain relief or if you have had a Caesarean section.

You may develop head, neck, back or leg pains for a few days after the birth as the effects of the drugs used – for example, for epidural or spinal anaesthetic – wear off. Tension headaches can also occur due to tiredness, and back and hip pain can result from being put in the lithotomy stirrups for stitching or a forceps or vacuum delivery. Neck pain may be due to prolonged pushing in the second stage of labour when your head is bent forwards on your chest, and this can be compounded by poor positioning during breastfeeding.

If you have had several babies or a very big baby, you may notice that the muscles which run down the middle of your abdomen on either side of your umbilicus (navel) protrude upwards and outwards when you attempt to sit upright. This is called divarification of the rectus sheath, and is due to the band of muscles becoming over-stretched in pregnancy and failing to firm up again afterwards. If left untreated it can lead to continuing back problems, because strength in the back is improved by well-toned abdominal muscles (see Postnatal exercises, page 197).

A similar problem which can cause significant discomfort is symphysis pubis pain, due to separation of the pad of cartilage in the middle of the pubic bones. If this has not been a problem during pregnancy, it may be initiated by prolonged positioning in stirrups during labour or afterwards for stitching.

Swollen ankles may initially become worse in the first few days after the birth as your kidneys struggle to cope with the excess fluid (see 'Private and personal', page 187). However, if you notice pain in your calf, especially when accompanied by a hot red area, you should notify your doctor or midwife as this could possibly be the beginnings of a blood clot in a blood vessel.

Tiredness may overwhelm you at times in the early days following the birth while you adjust to broken nights, yet sleep may be difficult because you feel so elated.

SELF-HELP

- **Massage** Gentle massage of the small of your back may ease aches which persist after epidural or spinal anaesthetic in labour. Upwards massage of your legs, using two hands, can temporarily reduce swelling of your ankles and calves, although it is likely to return when you stand upright, until the excess fluid has been excreted. It is important to note that leg massage should be avoided if you suspect problems with varicose veins or a blood clot. Head massage can be effective for relieving headaches. General all-over body massage is very relaxing and will facilitate sleep and rest.
- **Aromatherapy** Choose essential oils such as lavender, sandalwood, ylang ylang and rose for relaxation and relief of aches and pains. Marjoram is good for muscular back pain and cypress and juniper berry can be used in small amounts if you have varicose veins or swollen legs. Use four drops diluted in 5ml/1 teaspoon of carrier oil. Camomile may help you get to sleep – put two drops neat on your pillow.

Homeopathy following delivery

Unless otherwise stated, take one 30C tablet of the most appropriate remedy three times daily for three days.

- Arnica can be used after normal delivery, Caesarean section, forceps or vacuum delivery as well as breech delivery, to ease bruising and swelling. See the regimes give on pages 117 and 169.
- If you have bruises and soreness that are not helped by using arnica; you may also have lumps and bumps and possibly old injuries which feel tender – bellis perennis.
- If your wounds (episiotomy or Caesarean section) bleed freely with bright red blood which is slow to clot and are accompanied by burning pains; you have a great need for sympathy but are easily comforted; you feel worse when cold and in the evening or morning but better after sleep or when you have had a cold drink – phosphorus.

OTHER THERAPIES WHICH MAY HELP

For these therapies, refer to a qualified practitioner.

Reflexology can be effective in reducing neck and back tensions, or the rarely occurring severe headaches which some mothers develop after epidural anaesthetic (see Liz's story, opposite).

Osteopathy or **chiropractic**, for ongoing problems, will release tensions and realign the spinal column, which may have been affected by positions in labour, particularly the lithotomy stirrups. Most practitioners will advocate a routine postnatal treatment to correct any minor displacements which may have occurred during labour.

Cranial osteopathy is a very gentle means of easing aches and pains following the birth and can be particularly effective for ongoing problems which affect the whole of the spine.

Alexander technique can help you to correct your posture, which will have been affected by pregnancy, birth and breastfeeding. Specially adapted exercises may also help to firm up your abdominal muscles again if there is separation of the rectus sheath and can ease the discomfort of pubic pain.

Liz's story

Liz had given birth to Tom by forceps delivery two days before I was called to see her. She had had an epidural anaesthetic for the labour and a minor complication had occurred which caused her to have a severe ongoing headache after labour. The anaesthetist had been called to see her and was planning to perform a small procedure which would necessitate Liz remaining flat in bed for another 24 hours, in order to treat her headache. The midwives on the postnatal ward asked me to see Liz before the anaesthetist returned in case I could treat her more quickly. I performed reflexology on Liz's feet and found that the two big toes, which represent the head and neck, were very stiff and painful. I worked to release the stiffness and treat the headache and left Liz feeling more relaxed than she had been since the birth. Four hours later her headache had disappeared and Liz felt able to get up – she was so pleased that it meant she could go home early that she almost danced out of the ward!

Postnatal exercises

There are several exercises you can practise which will help in the process of recovery from pregnancy and birth. Try to make the effort to find time to do each set of exercises at least once daily and preferably more frequently, as it is easy to forget or become too busy or too tired. Some, such as pelvic floor exercises, should ideally be done regularly throughout pregnancy in preparation for labour, and then continued for the rest of your childbearing years! This will help to prevent some of the long-term effects of childbirth such as prolapse of your uterus in later life.

GENERAL EXERCISES

The following exercises will stimulate your general circulation:

- **Ankle circling** Sit or lie comfortably with your legs straight out in front of you. Keep your knees still and circle your ankles in one direction and then the other, about 12 times each way.
- **Leg tightening** Keeping your legs straight, pull your feet upwards, bringing you toes towards your nose and pressing the backs of your knees into the bed. Hold for three seconds, then relax, and repeat five times.

- **Deep breathing** Breathe in and out deeply and slowly, ensuring that your abdomen pushes outwards as you fill up your lungs with air and then inwards as you empty them; breathe five times, then return to normal breathing.
- Try not to spend long periods of time sitting or standing without changing your position, and avoid sitting with your legs crossed at all times. There is an increased risk of thrombosis (blood clots) in the first few days after delivery because the clotting ability of your blood has changed in order to prevent haemorrhage: crossing your legs temporarily restricts blood flow in your legs and increases this risk. Rest with your legs up on a stool when possible, and when in bed avoid crossing your ankles.

PELVIC FLOOR EXERCISES

These are the most important exercises any woman can do and you should try to do them whenever possible, but at least eight to ten times daily. Get into the habit of doing them when you are sitting down feeding your baby, when you are watching television or, later, when you are ironing or standing in the kitchen preparing meals. I remember once driving past two new mothers whom I had looked after – they were standing at the bus stop, giggling, and I found out later that they were doing their pelvic floor exercises together while they waited for the bus!

To perform the exercises, tighten up your anal sphincter (back passage) as if you are trying to prevent yourself from passing wind. Tighten your front muscles as if you are trying to stop yourself from passing urine and tighten your vaginal muscles as if you are squeezing your partner during sex. Pull up all three sets of muscles and hold for as long as possible, then relax and repeat up to ten times, first slowly and then quickly. Try not to hold your breath while you are doing the exercises. Although, after a few weeks, you can test out the effectiveness of your exercises by trying to stop passing urine while sitting on the toilet, you should not practise them all the time like this, as it will increase the risk of urinary infection from back-tracking of urine.

It can take several weeks to regain control of these muscles and initially you may feel no sensation at all. If you find yourself leaking urine when you cough, sneeze or laugh you need to continue to practise the exercises. If the problem persists, see your family doctor.

ABDOMINAL EXERCISES

- **Abdominal tightening** You can do this exercise from the very first day following the birth. Lying on your back with your knees bent, draw in your abdominal muscles and hold for a count of five, relax and repeat five times.
- **Pelvis tilts** Lying on your back with your knees bent, draw in your abdominal muscles as above, tighten the muscles of your buttocks and press the small of your back into the bed or floor. Hold for a count of five, relax and repeat five times on the first few days, increasing the number until you get to a maximum of 12 times daily by the end of the fourth week.

The following exercises should only be practised after the third day, on condition that you do not have separation of the abdominal muscles – if this is the case, speak to your midwife or physiotherapist about the safest and most appropriate exercises for you.

- **Curl-ups** Lie on your back, with your knees bent and pelvis tilted as above. Lift your head forwards and reach towards your knees with your hands, then lower your head back down. Repeat five times, then increase the number of repeats over a period of two weeks until you can manage 20 times. Later you can also practise this exercise by lifting your head and shoulders off the bed. On no account should you attempt to do full sit-up exercises as your back and abdominal muscles are not strong enough.
- **Knee rolling** Lie on your back, with your knees bent and pelvis tilted. Roll your two knees together to one side, keeping your shoulders straight – it may help to stretch both arms out straight on the bed or floor at right angles to your body. Bring your knees back to the middle, then roll them over to the other side. Repeat ten times, increasing to a maximum of 20 repetitions. It is important always to return your knees to the centre before rolling them to the other side.
- **Hip hitching** Lie on your back, with your left knee bent and right leg straight, with your right foot bent upwards. Push your right heel downwards to lengthen your right leg and pull in your abdominal muscles. Keeping your right knee straight, pull up your right hip towards

your ribs in order to shorten your right leg. Hold for a count of five, relax and repeat this five times on the right side, then repeat the entire procedure on the left side.

postnatal 'blues' and depression

Huge hormonal fluctuations occur in the early days following delivery, as the pregnancy hormones are expelled from your system with the placenta and those responsible for lactation increase. In about 50 per cent of new mothers, this can lead to third-day 'blues' as the balance of hormones shifts, the baby recovers from the birth and the physical adaptations of no longer being pregnant begin to take their full effect. You are very likely to feel weepy for no apparent reason, as well as tired, and you may feel a sense of anticlimax as all the attention from friends and family is directed away from you and towards your baby.

When to seek further advice

If you feel overwhelmingly depressed, anxious or obsessed with yourself or your baby, or if family or friends notice dramatic changes in your behaviour – such as being obsessed with hygiene, hyperactive or completely lethargic – you should contact your midwife or family doctor. Postnatal depression is relatively uncommon and is eminently treatable, but this depends on early recognition and prompt referral for specialist treatment.

SELF-HELP
- **Nutritional therapy** Ensuring a nourishing diet will help you to deal with the stresses and strains of adapting to parenthood, dealing with the tiredness, the sense of responsibility, establishment of breastfeeding and recovering from the pregnancy and labour. Eat plenty of foods which contain vitamins C and B as well as zinc, or take a good quality multivitamin and mineral supplement. Avoid stimulants such as tea,

coffee, cola, alcohol and too much chocolate. Eat adequate amounts of protein and at least four to five portions of fruit, vegetables or salad daily. Be sure to drink at least 3 litres of water or fruit juice every day.

- **Bach flower remedies** Walnut will protect you from outside influences (such as mothers-in-law!) and olive will relieve some of the tiredness. If you are a perfectionist and find it difficult to relinquish some of your daily chores, try vervain, or centaury if you insist on doing everything for yourself. Crab apple will reduce feelings of uncleanliness and elm is wonderful if you are overwhelmed by responsibility. If you become more seriously depressed, try mustard or gentian.

- **Herbal remedies** Camomile tea can be very calming and may help you to sleep when you are still 'on a high' from the birth. If you have access to fresh lavender, put a spray of the flowers and twigs under the running water as you prepare a bath, then lie back and enjoy a soak for a few minutes. Jasmine tea is particularly effective in cases of depression.

- **Aromatherapy** Good quality jasmine oil can be used in a massage or the bath; ylang ylang, neroli or rose are also lovely nurturing and relaxing oils. Use four drops, diluted in 5ml/1 teaspoon of carrier oil.

- **Relaxation techniques** Try some of the relaxation exercises which helped during pregnancy, such as SOS – Sigh Out Slowly – breathing and muscle relaxation (see page 66), especially if you become very stressed.

- **Yoga** or **Tai Chi** As your baby gets older and you have more time available, you may gain benefit from attending classes: some areas have classes specifically for new mothers where a crèche is also available.

Homeopathy

Take one 30C tablet of the most appropriate remedy three times daily for three days.

- If you find yourself weeping at night, are exhausted, apathetic, sad and lack appetite; you feel worse if given sympathy or if you are touched, but better from writing things down – China.

- If you are tearful, sigh a lot and feel trapped by having to care for your baby; you are unable to sleep after breastfeeding your baby, feel worse in the afternoon or if you have a headache, and can become very excitable on the occasions when your dejection lifts – cimicifuga.

- If you have difficulty crying and prefer to be on your own to do so; your moods may alternate from deep depression to inappropriate hilarity and are worse in the late morning or if you are consoled; you eat well but appear to be losing weight – natrum mur.
- If you constantly break down in tears, especially when spoken to, yet your moods are changeable; you feel worse in the evening or in a stuffy room, but better in company and when given sympathy; your memory and attention span are poor and you may feel you are going insane – pulsatilla.
- If you cry involuntarily for no real reason, you are indifferent to your baby and family and feel empty; you are worse in the evening or in the open air but feel better if you get some exercise or when you are alone, although you may dread being left on your own; you are restless and perspire easily and feel you must scream or do something desperate – sepia.

OTHER THERAPIES WHICH MAY HELP

For these therapies, refer to a qualified practitioner.

Acupuncture or **acupressure** can be used to rebalance energies, which is especially important at this time when so many physical, emotional and spiritual upheavals are occurring in your life. **Shiatsu** practitioners call the childbearing experience one of the significant 'Gateways of Change' in which it is vital to ensure rest, adequate nutrients and appropriate balance of Yin and Yang energies.

Alexander technique classes can be relaxing and may assist in relieving many of the minor physical symptoms related to the postnatal period which can contribute to 'blues' and depression.

Hypnotherapy can ease you through some of the longer-term emotional problems which can exacerbate and prolong postnatal depression.

Massage from a qualified practitioner, on a regular basis, will have cumulative effects that can produce long-term benefits.

Cranial osteopathy is relaxing and releases tensions which contribute to emotional disturbances; osteopathy or chiropractic can also help.

Reflexology is also useful, as a regular treatment, simply for relaxation, as well as for dealing with the physical problems which may persist.

Baby problems

This book has covered conditions which may affect you during pregnancy, labour or in the immediate postnatal period, and the ways in which complementary therapies may help. It is not the intention here to explore in depth the potential of complementary medicine for treating problems that your baby may develop, as serious conditions can develop rapidly in small babies and any concerns you have should always be referred to your family doctor.

The aims of the care your baby receives in the first few weeks from your midwife, doctor or health visitor are to ensure that s/he is adapting normally to independent life outside your uterus. Initially these adaptations focus on establishing adequate respiration and circulation. Several changes occur in the baby's circulation, heart and lungs in the first 24 hours following birth. During foetal life the baby requires a greater number of red blood cells to help push oxygen around his/her body. Many of these are not needed after birth and are broken down by the baby's liver and excreted. However, it is common for the liver, which is still immature, to be slow to complete this process and this is one of the reasons why newborn babies often develop a temporary jaundice (yellowing of the skin). In most cases this is normal, but your baby will be observed closely by the midwife or doctor to ensure that no complications develop.

Your baby is susceptible to infection in the early weeks until s/he develops his/her own immunity – one of the best ways to help this along is to breastfeed, and of course to pay attention to normal hygiene. A newborn baby's stools are initially black (as the intestines expel extra cells used in foetal life), then brown, then yellow, until s/he starts eating solid foods. Your baby's temperature-regulating mechanism is also not well developed and you need to consider appropriate clothing to ensure that s/he is neither too hot nor too cold.

While most babies adapt to life as independent beings without complications, minor problems can occasionally occur which, although not in need of medical attention, can cause you anxiety and worry. Remember that crying is your baby's way of communicating something to you – whether or not s/he is hungry, thirsty, wet, dirty, hot, cold, bored, in need of a cuddle or in pain. Gradually you will learn to interpret the different cries, but in the first few months you should never ignore your baby's crying as it may be indicative of either a minor disorder or something more serious. Here are a few examples of conditions which can easily be resolved by using specific strategies from complementary medicine.

colic and digestive conditions

Some babies are naturally very colicky or 'windy' and suffer spasmodic abdominal discomfort as a result of air trapped in the intestines. They may have a lot of wind during or immediately after feeding, which may be passed out rectally or by 'burping', or cause abdominal distension and pain. Constipation can occur in a few babies or, perhaps more commonly, diarrhoea. A few babies may be affected by the foods you eat while breastfeeding, although this should not normally be a problem if you eat everything in moderation. You may find that any change in your diet after returning home from hospital triggers colic temporarily.

SELF-HELP

- **Massage** Gentle abdominal massage in a clockwise direction can stimulate movement of the intestines and therefore treat both constipation and colic. Use your fingertips and a tiny drop of baby oil to work in a firm circular motion around the whole of your baby's tummy. If s/he has diarrhoea, the massage should be anticlockwise to slow down movement of the gut, although you need to be sure that there is no infection present as diarrhoea may actually be the body's way of eliminating it.

- **Aromatherapy** As a general rule, it is best to avoid essential oils for your baby in the early months, but *one drop* of a good quality camomile oil can be very effective in resolving constipation and colic. Add this to 5ml/1 teaspoon of carrier oil and gently massage the abdomen in a clockwise direction. Camomile has a very high concentration of a particular type of chemical which is anti-spasmodic and so will reduce griping pains.

- **Herbal remedies** Similarly, camomile can be used – make up a cup of camomile tea with boiling water and allow it to cool. Give your baby 10ml/2 teaspoons of the tea on a sterilized spoon, twice daily until the symptoms subside. This remedy can be effective for constipation, colic or diarrhoea.

- **Reflexology** Gently but firmly massage the arches (insteps) of your baby's feet (see fig. 4, page 209) in a clockwise direction if s/he has colic or constipation. If your baby has loose stools, perhaps as a result of something you have eaten if you are breastfeeding, you could perform massage to the arches of the feet in an anticlockwise direction to slow down the movement of the gut. You can use some baby oil or an aromatherapy carrier oil such as sweet almond to help your fingers slide over the skin. However, if there is a change in either the colour or odour of the stools, which could indicate that your baby has developed a gastric infection such as gastroenteritis, you should seek advice from your midwife or family doctor and refrain from performing the foot massage until you are sure that no infection is present. This is so that the baby is able to eliminate the infection.
- **Bach flower remedies** A few drops of Rescue Remedy can be effective in calming your baby if s/he is extremely fretful, although this will not of course deal with the cause. If you are becoming distressed, anxious or exasperated by constant crying, four drops neat on your tongue will help you too!

Homeopathy

Place a few granules of the 6C potency of the most appropriate remedy on your baby's tongue, as required.

- If your baby has colic with a tense, hard, bloated abdomen, screams and draws up his/her legs, which is worse in the evening; s/he vomits greenish vomit or curdled milk, may have green/yellow diarrhoea and a red face; you will probably be breastfeeding your baby but may be feeling angry about something – chamomilla.
- If your baby is irritable, constantly straining to have his/her bowels open, without success, with a lot of wind, all of which is worse in the morning; you will be breastfeeding but may have eaten spicy food or drunk too much tea, coffee or cola – nux vomica.
- If there is colic with empty burping, sickness and lots of saliva; your baby does not like to be moved and the problem is worse after feeding; you may be breastfeeding but are experiencing feelings of anger or frustration – ipecacuanha.

- If constipation is present with a large, hard, knotty stool that is difficult to expel despite constant urging; your baby is irritable, yet worse when picked up to be consoled or when hot; s/he may refuse your milk and there is perspiration on his/her head during feeding – silica.

OTHER THERAPIES WHICH MAY HELP
For these therapies, refer to a qualified practitioner.
Chiropractic was used in a large trial in Denmark, which found that babies suffering colic could be treated promptly and effectively with this therapy; **osteopathy** may also help.

sticky eyes

Your baby does not cry tears for the first few weeks after birth and occasionally the tear ducts become blocked, leading to a condition known as sticky eyes. A few babies will develop infection in the eyes which will need to be adequately treated to avoid long-term problems, but most cases of sticky eyes resolve relatively quickly without complications.

When to seek further advice
If the stickiness in your baby's eyes persists for more than a few days, or if it becomes very pus-like in consistency or changes colour, consult your midwife, health visitor or family doctor.

SELF-HELP
- **Herbal remedies** Use cooled camomile tea as an eye wash – gently wipe with cottonwool soaked in camomile tea, working from the inner aspect of each eye outwards, to remove any stickiness. This will help to reduce inflammation and act as an antiseptic.
- **Colostrum** The highly nutritious milk present in your breasts in the early days before the milk supply becomes properly established is called

colostrum and is packed with anti-infective properties. If your baby has sticky eyes, try gently squeezing out some of the colostrum from your nipples directly into his/her eyes.

Homeopathy

Place a few granules of the 6C potency of the most appropriate remedy on your baby's tongue three times daily for three days.

- If there is profuse watering from the eyes with the lids swollen and red; the problem is worse in a cold wind and in the light, and your baby is restless and anxious – aconite.
- If there is thick mucus being discharged from the eyes, which are sensitive to light and the lids are stuck together, red, swollen and appear to itch; your baby may sleep well at night but cry all day – lycopodium.
- If the eyes appear gritty, watery and mucusy, with heavy twitching and sore-looking eyelids; your baby seems not to want too much physical contact and the right eye is especially badly affected – natrum mur.
- If there is a thick, yellow, purulent mucus discharge from the eyes, especially the left; the lids are stuck together, red, swollen and itching, worse in the evening and better in fresh cold air; your baby wants to be carried around gently and, if older, will be clingy and dependent – pulsatilla.

minor traumas and irritations

Mild skin rashes are common in newborn babies as a result of heat, blocked sweat glands and occasionally when faeces are left on the skin around the anus. 'Nappy rash' is usually preventable by frequent changing to dry napkins and ensuring that your baby does not stay in nappies that are soiled with faeces, but it can also occur due to thrush infection acquired as your baby travelled down the birth canal.

Babies delivered by forceps, vacuum or following a prolonged and difficult labour may have bruises on their heads, or an abnormal swelling which is either fluid (oedema) or more severe bruising (haematoma). They may also be more fretful than babies delivered normally, possibly due to pressure inside their heads. Some complementary therapists such as cranial osteopaths believe that babies delivered by forceps are more prone to thumb-sucking, as they subconsciously and spontaneously attempt to relieve this pressure (see Caesarean section and forceps delivery, page 169).

SELF-HELP
- **Bach flower remedies** Rescue Remedy cream is a gentle cream suitable for babies who have skin rashes and can be applied carefully to the relevant areas. If you apply the cream to the buttocks and are using disposable nappies, you should wipe away any excess before putting on a dry nappy, as it may interfere with the nappy lining's mechanism of drawing fluid away from the skin and can exacerbate the problem of nappy rash.
- **Herbal remedies** Calendula (marigold) cream can be applied to any sore areas, with the same proviso as above. Severe nappy rash may be eased by washing the skin in cooled camomile tea to reduce the inflammation, or by applying moist, cooled camomile teabags to the buttocks while the baby sleeps. Exposing the skin to the air afterwards will also help.
- **Aromatherapy** Two drops of tea tree oil mixed into a 50ml tub of water-based cream will be effective in treating thrush which develops as a rash on the buttocks; alternatively, a commercial version may be available.

Homeopathy
Unless otherwise stated, place a few granules of the 6C potency of the most appropriate remedy on your baby's tongue three times daily for three days.
- Arnica cream is the most appropriate means of dealing with bruising, but should not be applied to broken skin.
- If arnica clears up the skin irritation or bruise but a lump or bump remains – bellis perennis.
- If arnica does not resolve the bruise – sulphuric acidum.

OTHER THERAPIES WHICH MAY HELP

For these therapies, refer to a qualified practitioner.

Cranial osteopathy is a gentle treatment that has been shown in research to be extremely effective in calming babies who are fretful following forceps delivery, as well as older babies who are found to be hyperactive.

Self-help reflexology and acupressure points

fig. 1 hand and wrist

upper surface _____

Li4 acupressure point:

in webbing between thumb and forefinger

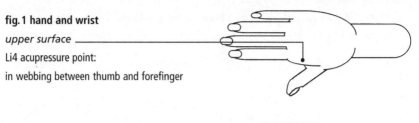

palmar surface, inner aspect of wrist _____

P6 acupressure point: measure 3 finger-widths

from wrist crease

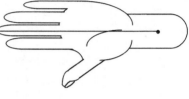

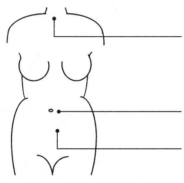

fig. 2 abdomen

CV22 acupressure point:

at base of throat, at junction

of collar bones

umbilicus

CV6 acupressure point:

3 finger-widths below umbilicus

fig. 3 head

GV20 acupressure point: _____

on very top, middle of head

B2 acupressure point: _____

just below ridge of bone over eyes

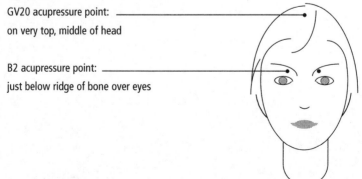

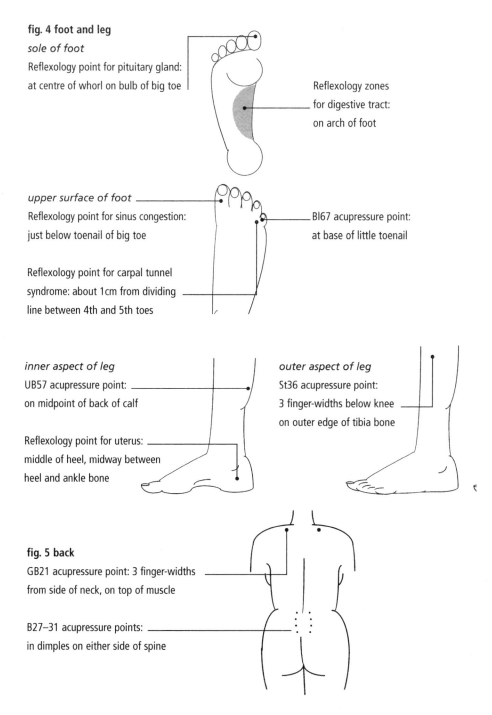

fig. 4 foot and leg

sole of foot
Reflexology point for pituitary gland:
at centre of whorl on bulb of big toe

Reflexology zones
for digestive tract:
on arch of foot

upper surface of foot
Reflexology point for sinus congestion:
just below toenail of big toe

Bl67 acupressure point:
at base of little toenail

Reflexology point for carpal tunnel
syndrome: about 1cm from dividing
line between 4th and 5th toes

inner aspect of leg
UB57 acupressure point:
on midpoint of back of calf

outer aspect of leg
St36 acupressure point:
3 finger-widths below knee
on outer edge of tibia bone

Reflexology point for uterus:
middle of heel, midway between
heel and ankle bone

fig. 5 back
GB21 acupressure point: 3 finger-widths
from side of neck, on top of muscle

B27–31 acupressure points:
in dimples on either side of spine

Useful addresses

Osteopathy
General Osteopathic Council
Osteopathy House
176 Tower Bridge Road
London SE1 3LU

Chiropractic
General Chiropractic Council
344–345 Gray's Inn Road
London WC1X 3XX

Homeopathy
Faculty of Homeopathy
2 Powis Place
London WC1N 3HT
*Trains doctors in homeopathy
and can direct you to doctors who
are also homeopaths; linked to
the Royal London Homeopathic
Hospital in Queen's Square,
London WC1N 2LT, one of five
NHS homeopathic hospitals.*

Society of Homeopaths
2 Artizan Road
Northampton NN1 4HU
*Main organization for the training
of non-medically qualified (lay)
homeopaths; holds a register of
practitioners.*

Ainsworth's Homeopathic Pharmacy
38 New Cavendish Street
London W1M 7LH
Homeopathic remedies by mail order.

Acupuncture
British Acupuncture Council
Park House
206–208 Latimer Road
London W10 6RE

Medical herbalism
National Institute of Medical Herbalists
56 Longbrook Street
Exeter EX4 4AH

Aromatherapy
Aromatherapy Organizations Council
3 Latymer Close
Braybrooke
Market Harborough LE16 8LL
*Holds a register of approved schools
of aromatherapy; can direct you to
individual schools which hold their
own registers of practitioners.*

Reflexology
Association of Reflexologists
27 Old Gloucester Street
London WC1N 3XX

British School of Reflex Zone Therapy
23 Marsh Hall
Talisman Way
Wembley Park HA9 8JJ

Massage

British Massage Therapy Council

17 Rymers Lane

Oxford OX4 3J

Shiatsu

The Shiatsu Society

Barber House

Storeys Bar Road

Fengate

Peterborough PE1 5YS

Hypnotherapy

British Society of Clinical Hypnotherapists

229a Sussex Gardens

Lancaster Gate

London W2 2RL

British Society of Medical and Dental

Hypnosis

17 Keppel View

Kimberworth

Rotherham S61 2AR

Alexander technique

Society of Teachers of the Alexander

Technique

20 London House

266 Fulham Road

London SW10 9EL

Nutritional therapy

British Association of Nutritional Therapists

27 Old Gloucester Street

London WC1N 3XX

Yoga

British Wheel of Yoga

46 Rectory Road

Upton on Severn WR8 0QG

**Other organizations
and services**

Complementary Therapies in Maternity Care

National Forum

c/o Denise Tiran (Chair)

School of Health

University of Greenwich

Avery Hill Campus

Bexley Road

Eltham

London SE9 2UG

*Multidisciplinary professional
organization for health professionals
involved in using complementary
medicine for pregnancy and childbirth;
is developing a national register
of maternity complementary therapy
services.*

Zita West Pregnancy Products

Tel: 0870 166 8899

Website: www.zitawest.com

*Mail order natural medicine products
specially for pregnancy, labour and the
early postnatal days, based on up-to-
date research.*

index

Acknowledgements

I would like to thank all the expectant mothers whom I have treated in my clinic at Queen Mary's Hospital, Sidcup in Kent, UK, for the privilege of being able to assist in making their pregnancies and labours more satisfying and comfortable through the use of a range of complementary therapies. My gratitude is also extended to the midwives and obstetricians at Queen Mary's, who are so supportive of my work. I would also like to acknowledge my colleagues and students at the University of Greenwich, from whom I continue to learn while sharing my own knowledge of complementary medicine.

I would like to thank my editor, Jane O'Shea, at Quadrille, for guiding and supporting me through the energy-consuming process of writing this book. Thanks also are extended to Sarah Widdicombe, copy editor, who very patiently dealt with all the queries arising during the various stages of production.

Most of all, I would like to thank my wonderful son, Adam, aged 11, who has sat through many an evening without being able to talk to me while I finished the writing. Adam was born at home after a 24 hour labour during which I used various complementary therapies – he continues to enjoy their benefits whenever he can persuade me to find some time to pamper him!